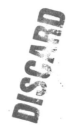
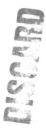

CARRYING THE HEART

CARRYING
THE
HEART

EXPLORING THE WORLDS
WITHIN US

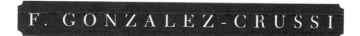

F. GONZALEZ-CRUSSI

KAPLAN

PUBLISHING

New York

This publication is designed to provide accurate and authoritative information in regard to the subject matter covered. It is sold with the understanding that the publisher is not engaged in rendering legal, accounting, or other professional service. If legal advice or other expert assistance is required, the services of a competent professional should be sought.

Published by Kaplan Publishing, a division of Kaplan, Inc.
1 Liberty Plaza, 24th Floor
New York, NY 10006

Printed in the United States of America

Library of Congress Cataloging-in-Publication Data

Gonzalez-Crussi, F.
Carrying the heart : exploring the worlds within us / by F. González-Crussí.
    p. ; cm.
ISBN 978-1-60714-072-6
1. Human physiology--Popular works. 2. Human anatomy--Popular works.
I. Title.
[DNLM: 1. Philosophy, Medical--Essays. 2. History of Medicine--Essays.
3. Physicians--history--Essays. W 61 G643c 2009]
    QP38.G657 2009
    612--dc22
                                    2009007195

10 9 8 7 6 5 4 3 2 1

Kaplan Publishing books are available at special quantity discounts to use for sales promotions, employee premiums, or educational purposes. Please email our Special Sales Department to order or for more information at *kaplanpublishing@kaplan.com*, or write to Kaplan Publishing, 1 Liberty Plaza, 24th Floor, New York, NY 10006.

Contents

Foreword

OR A VERY LONG time, the body was represented as a closed object, astonishing in its capacity for exquisitely coordinated actions—and in its admirable external proportions—but the interior of which remained forever sealed off. Here resided the arcane, impenetrable, seemingly unknowable secret of life. Then, through the unflagging, centuries long toiling of medical scientists, the mystery was resolved into a maze of living tubes, pipes, wires, valves, flasks, cogs, and wheels, with which the body manages to draw energy from the outer environment and feed it into its amazingly complex structure. Thus its functioning is ensured.

As valuable as the scientific analysis undoubtedly is, it brought with it an untoward effect: doing away with the innumerable symbolic meanings of the body, divested it of all moral value, and reduced it to the status of a machine. Modern medicine performs amazing procedures, such as organ transplants, genetic modifications, in vitro fertilization, and so on. But the human body is treated like a machine that may be tinkered with: its components are removed and exchanged, its electrical circuits reconnected, and its obstructed pipes unclogged. The body is "a wonderful machine," as many a commonplace puts it, but it is still considered a mechanical contrivance and nothing more. And note that in these trite sayings, the body is habitually compared to a machine, not a machine to the body. This shows well the order of priorities that rule most present-day thinking.

The contemporary anthropologist David Le Breton has pointed out that the fundamental human unity has been fragmented: a human being is no longer thought of as an "incarnate" entity—that is, a being linked indissolubly and for the whole duration of his or her life to a body. Instead a duality is posited: humanity versus corporeality, with a body on one side, and a human subject on the other. In the 21st century, medicine looks after the body with meticulous (sometimes excessive) conscientiousness but coolly brushes aside the human dimension, so that the patient as a unique human subject is not taken into consideration. Professional medical attention could not be more intensely focused upon the disease process, yet it could not be more perfunctory in its view of the man or the woman who suffers from it.

The role of the patient is to submit passively and surrender trustingly into the hands of health care professionals. They, of course, look at the body abstracted from the individualized, suffering human being. In this objectifying schema, the patient cannot possibly imagine what is happening inside his body. He does not have the necessary knowledge, and it is his sad lot merely to repine under the crush of evil forces that he does not understand and is fated never to understand. Under this set of circumstances, now all too common in Western societies, the sick are not encouraged to participate in their own healing.

All of this has been a subject of concern for numerous writers. The mass of commentary that these problems have elicited is overwhelming. It is not my purpose to add to this enormous quantity. Rather, I thought it appropriate to increase the public's awareness of the body's insides. By this, I do not mean the objective facts of anatomy, for most educated people today have a general, if limited, understanding of the body's parts and functions. I mean the history, the symbolism, the reflections, the many ideas, serious or fanciful, and even the romance and lore with which the inner organs have been surrounded historically. I've arranged the chapters much like an anatomy book, with each section devoted to an organ system but addressing mostly nontechnical aspects of the organs. By showing the elaborate effort with which the creative imagination has embroidered the body's interiority throughout the ages and across all cultures, I hope to underscore the significance of the symbolic dimension of our lives, which current medical techno-science largely disregards.

The body is *not* a machine. Unlike a machine, it has a faculty of imagination that surrounds it like a permanent, indelible halo. The imaginary keeps coming back, stubbornly, despite all efforts to suppress it. Everyone will make his or her own representation of the body's interiority. For man's life is as much a life of organic physiology as it is one of relations, representations, symbols, dreams, and imaginations. Mind you, these are not idle, ineffectual, and useless illusions. The so-called fantasies constitute the point of departure for our interaction with the world, and their power is in evidence everywhere. The well-known and mighty placebo effect stands as a compelling testimony to the great force of symbol and imagination on the body. Thus, in this book the reader will find reference to the fact that an imaginary upset or a mental representation perceived as negative—for instance, a disappointment—can trigger severe organic damage to the heart, and even death.

Disease is largely a construction of society; therefore it is experienced differently by people in different communities and during different epochs. Accordingly, the reader will find here reference to historical concepts that granted the stomach a higher place in the processing of emotions and the origination of diseases than we are willing to concede. Curiously, others believed that the rectum was the preeminent organ in determining our health and longevity. For it has been a peculiarity of our mental representations of the body to create a hierarchy of the internal organs. Some revered the brain as supreme. Others elevated the heart to the highest dignity, while reviling the intestines, conduits for the elimination of refuse. As often happens, an unschooled, earthy rustic was the voice of good sense. In Miguel de Cervantes Saavedra's *Don Quixote*, Sancho Panza, the mad knight's good squire, declares, "It is not the heart that carries the tripes, but the tripes that carry the heart." In other words, our organs are mutually interdependent, and it is a fact that our highest-minded impulses depend on those functions that our fancy labels vulgar, crude, or insignificant.

The imaginary representation of the body is but one aspect of the flow of symbols that informs and pervades human life. This symbolic movement is a very powerful force. *Carrying the Heart* was written in the hope that one day medicine will find ways to use this force to potentiate the benefits of its therapies, thereby transforming the patient from a passive entity into an active participant in his own cure.

Digestive

The Reign of the Stomach

Well over fivescore years ago (here I feel compelled inwardly to exclaim, "Who would have believed it!"), as I was growing up in a proletarian neighborhood of the then slow-paced and relatively tranquil City of Mexico (qualifications, these, that quicken in me a still stronger reaction of stupefied disbelief), it was not uncommon to hear people say that their moral crises were experienced as impacts on a specific anatomical site. This somatic focal point, this "shock organ," so to speak, of their psychological storms, was the stomach. Anyone who received a disagreeable surprise, learned bad news, had an altercation, or suffered any of the many forms of stress to which the poor everywhere seem more vulnerable than the affluent, felt the effects of personal misfortune in the upper abdomen.

Thus, my mother, oppressed by financial want and under the duress of her creditors' inflexibility, translated her monthly anxiety about not being able to make ends meet into a concrete gastric sensation. The weight of her woes somehow gravitated upon her person; not on her shoulders, as the trite metaphor would have it, but, in a very literal sense, on a restricted zone of the abdomen, which she would point at and say: "*aquí, en la boca del estómago*" ("right here, in the stomach's mouth"). "The stomach's mouth" seemed to me at the time an unsophisticated expression. In my callowness, I thought of it somewhat contemptuously as the utterance of the unlearned, who were ignorant of the basic rudiments of human anatomy and naive enough to think that the stomach could be the nucleus, hub, and pivot of the emotions. May God have forgiven my youthful impudence. Subsequently, I learned how ignorant and mistaken I was.

The fact is, the stomach's mouth is a term of ancient lineage: *stoma*, said the ancient Greeks, who used it profusely in their medical treatises. The Romans referred to it as *cardia*, because of its proximity to the heart, and to this day it remains the technical name of the entrance orifice, or mouth, of the stomach. Galen, the renowned Greek physician of the second century, pointed out that the cardia of the stomach is richly endowed with nerves and possesses a great sensitivity, thereby being able to cause systemic disorders that are manifested through the heart, such as syncope, suffocation, lethargy, spasms, melancholia, and others. Therefore, the Galenic school maintained that many disorders attributed to the heart in reality come from the cardia of the stomach. Ancient writings that include the term most often refer to the stomach, not to the heart, leading to confusion in ill-informed or incompetent modern translators.[1]

The preeminence of the stomach in the body was recognized by the ancients. In a well-known passage of the ancient historian Livy's *History of Rome* (II, 32) we are told that Menenius Agrippa, consul in the year 503 B.C., referred to the importance of the stomach in a parable that served his political ends. What happened was the following: The common people, indignant at the uneven distribution of power and complaining of the abuses they suffered from the senatorial party, staged a revolt and left the city. Fear and tension reigned in Rome, lest the rebels might wish to vindicate their rights by force; but the rebels, too, were much afraid of the violence that their adversaries might inflict upon them. At this juncture, the senators deputized Menenius Agrippa to parley with the rebels, who sympathized with him because he had come from their own ranks. He knew how to talk to them and told them ("in the rugged style of those far-off days," says Livy), a fable about the stomach, or "the belly," that convinced them to put down their arms and return to the city.

The stomach, goes the story, was looked at askance by the rest of the bodily parts because it seemed to do nothing but enjoy the sustenance that they brought to him. Resentful, the hands declared that they would no longer present food to the mouth; the mouth, that thenceforward it was not going to open to admit any foodstuffs; the teeth and the jaws, that they would refuse to grind anything that the mouth received. All the bodily parts resented the fact that the stomach merely accepted the booty that all of them worked hard to procure. But, alas, while they were trying to subdue the stomach by starvation, it became clear that they too would waste away for lack of nutriment. They realized that the stomach is no idle poltroon but has its own important function that it must fulfill for the common good. This function is to transform the rough ingesta into the nourishing fluid that is then absorbed in the intestine and distributed via the circulating blood to all the parts of the organism.

The stomach, said Menenius Agrippa to the insurgents, was the senate or the patrician class; the bodily parts were the rebellious plebeians. And just as the city could not survive without plebeians, the latter could not live without the patricians. Presumably, this mediocre parable convinced the untutored plebs to return to the city and to their original trades. Shakespeare, who repeats the fable in *Coriolanus*, has the stomach lecturing to the rest of the organs (whom he addresses as "my incorporate friends") about the importance of his function, which is

> That I receive the general food at first
> Which you do live upon; and fit it is
> Because I am the store-house and the shop
> Of the whole body. But, if you do remember,
> I send it through the rivers of your blood
> Even to the court, the heart, to th'seat o' th'brain;
> And through the cranks and offices of man,
> The strongest nerves and small inferior veins
> From me receive that natural competency
> Whereby they live ...
>
> (Act I, scene 1, 130–139)

Because of its alleged leading role in joy and adversity, some physicians of the past did not hesitate in making the stomach the seat of the soul, a title it long disputed to the heart and the brain; and it was specifically the cardia, the mouth of the stomach, that was thought to be the place where the principle of life and strength resided. The ancients called it "the king of viscera," and Hippocrates said that it was, in the microcosm of the body, what the sea was in the macrocosm of the world: an entity with the faculty of giving to all and taking from all. (As the ancients put it: *Maris habens facultatem qui omnibus dat et ab omnibus accipit.*)[1]

In the Middle Ages, the French surgeon and royal physician Henri de Mondeville (CA. 1260–CA. 1325) referred to the stomach as "the most principal and noble organ," whose orderly function determined the integrity of the whole organism. The Italian physician Alessandro Benedetti (1452–1512), in a similar context, referred to the stomach's mouth as "father of the family," since the health of the whole body was subordinate to the cardia's functioning normally. Melancholia, a form of insanity characterized by depression, was supposed to be the unfortunate consequence of a deficient working of the gastric cardia, in contrast to the psychiatric illness known as fury, or mania, the origin of which could be traced to a diseased brain.[2]

Paracelsus (CA. 1493–1541), that strange personage of the history of medicine (whose true, splendid name was Theophrastus Philippus Aureolus Bombastus von Hohenheim), was alchemist, physician, and unorthodox thinker with a bent for mysticism and esotericism, and became, in the words of the respected British historian Roy Porter,[3] "the scourge of the medical Establishment" of his time. Welding together spiritual and vital forces with chemical principles, Paracelsus tried to explain the living process and was among the first to envisage disease as a chemical disturbance of the organism—albeit through a fog of recondite, impenetrable notions. He proposed the existence of an arcane vital principle that he called *arche*, or *archeus*. Difficult as it may be to make sense of his abstruse writings, the concept of archeus seems to overlap in some respects with the idea of the soul, and to this mysterious entity, he gave the stomach as place of residence.

One of his most devoted followers was Joan Baptista van Helmont (1579–1644), from Vilvoorde, in the Spanish Netherlands (now Belgium); he is credited with important early insights in biochemistry and the identification of carbon dioxide, and is said to have invented the word *gas*. Following the teachings of Paracelsus, van Helmont proposed the existence of a life force on which depended the natural reparative processes of the organism, not unlike the Paracelsian archeus. Like his mentor, he thought that this force, which exerted dominion over most corporeal processes, was inseparable from the stomach.

Thus, the stomach long occupied a supreme hierarchical position in Western medical thought. This organ exerted a sort of physiological principate through an officious gastric mouth that had the wisdom to open to receive the nourishment, and to close to impede noxious "vapors" or effluences from reaching other parts of the body. As late as the beginning of the 19th century, a colorful physician and veteran of the Napoleonic wars, François Joseph Victor Broussais (1772–1838), following the example of the ancients, called the stomach "king of the economy" and elaborated a peculiar medical doctrine that for a while enjoyed immense popularity. He proposed that there were no such things as individual diseases, but that all types of pathology were inflammations or irritations centered upon the gastrointestinal system. Inflammation could be transmitted to other organs via the nervous system or through other mechanisms, and thus the symptoms could be quite variable, but ultimately their seat was in the stomach, whose mucosal lining was uniquely susceptible to inflammation. Phrased differently, there was but one disease: gastroenteritis. As one of Broussais's followers put it, the stomach "is and forever shall be, the key of pathology."

However, more than a century before Broussais began practicing medicine, a mounting opposition to the hypothetical reign of the stomach had already started. Thomas Bartholin (1616–1680), a Dutch anatomist who produced the first comprehensive description of the lymphatic system, opposed the concept of a preeminent stomach with arguments that today make us smile. If the stomach is the seat of the soul, he wondered, does it mean that gluttons and all who manifest a voracious appetite have more soul than their leaner fellows or those generally indifferent to the pleasures of the table? Furthermore, the gastric cardia admits and stores impure food, without this having any discernible effect on the soul. Nor is the soul damaged by performers at circuses and country fairs who lower swords and knives into the stomach.

The stomach began to be looked at objectively, like any other organ. Regarded in this light, the stomach presents itself to our eyes as a muscular-membranous bag whose form is considerably modified according to its tonicity and the amount of its contents.

The "classical" stomach shape as seen in cadavers, says a venerable French treatise of anatomy, is that of "a bagpipe, flattened from front to back and directed transversely or rather obliquely from left to right, from front to back, and from up to down, with two curvatures of unequal size: the large curvature above, and the smaller below."[4] When one opens the abdomen during a cadaver dissection, this organ is largely hidden by the ribs on the left side, and on the right by the liver, which covers a good part of its anterior face. In the cadaver, the stomach has lost its tonicity and is flaccid, its lower portion resting upon the transverse colon and its "meso" (peritoneal support sheet), which form a kind of bed for it.

Matter-of-fact descriptions of this kind mean to divest the stomach of its mystery; in the name of science, the viscus is ignominiously demoted from princely ruler of the organism and seat of the soul to mere muscular-membranous bag—comparable, at best, to a bagpipe. Yet the variability of its morphology, to say nothing of its astounding functions, hints that a restitution of its wonder is not far away. The student of anatomy is soon made aware that the stomach's form and volume vary greatly among living human beings: impressively large in guzzlers and gormandizers; of very modest dimensions in abstemious and self-mortifying ascetics; shrunk and compacted in the hypertonic type, more common in the athletic and robust, whose stomach resembles a cornucopia (surely, a horn of abundance beats a bagpipe!); shaped like the letter *J* in the normal or "orthonic" type; piteously flabby and elongated down to the pelvis in the atonic type; and so on.

But if the gastric shape varies with the individual among human beings, what a dazzling kaleidoscope turns up when comparisons are made between species! Fishes have their stomach almost at their outer surface. As a 19th-century English naturalist put it, in a prose style that unfortunately has been banned from today's scientific literature:

> They are all stomach, like the larvae of other species, and are chiefly intent upon the gratification of their voracious appetites. All other sense seems to be absorbed in this. No soft sounds to charm their ears are heard in the silent deep. No roaring of lions, or other fierce animals, to excite their alarm. They are dumb, because they have no lungs nor larynx; and so they should be, as they are also deaf. Their huge eyeballs, what can they see to engage their attention but their prey in the vast dark deep, clouded with mud, or the ever-moving sands? You see, therefore, that all their senses but that of hunger are obtuse.[5]

In some lemurs (primitive primates of the Lemuridae family), the stomach is globular; in the porcupine it has three pockets; in the pika, or mouse hare (tailless rabbitlike mammal), it is crescentic; in the wombat, an Australian marsupial, it is pear shaped; in ruminating quadrupeds, it is four chambered and acquires a singular appearance; but in all mammals, the stomach is membranous. In many birds, especially the graminivorous (grass feeding), there is a glandular stomach, but there is also what is called the gizzard: a globular, compacted receptacle endowed with enormously thick, muscular walls, while its inner membranous lining is coriaceous, wrinkled, and hard, to protect it from lacerations, for here are stored the pebbles and gravel that serve these birds as organs of mastication, given their lack of teeth and jaws. Says our English naturalist, "If you deprive those gallinaceous birds of their pebbles, you might as well deprive them of their food, or deprive a ruminating quadruped of all its teeth; they will languish and starve in both cases."[6]

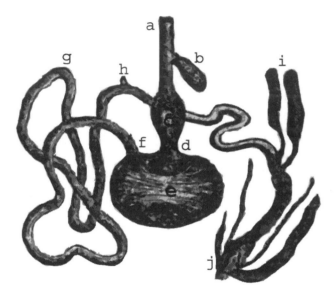

Fig. 1 Avian (gallinaceous birds) gastrointestinal tract. From Robert E. Grant's "Lectures in Comparative Anatomy" (*The Lancet*, 1833–4): (a) esophagus, (b) esophageal pouch or "crop," (c) glandular stomach, (d) cardial extremity, (e) heavily muscular gizzard, (f) pyloric extremity, (g) small intestine, (h) remnant of vitelline duct, (i) pair of ceca, (j) cloaca.

However, we are not graminivorous birds. We do not have a gizzard, but share with the birds of prey a relatively thin, membranous stomach. This is characteristic of vultures as well as of wolves, dogs, lions, and carnivores in general. For, make no mistake, our meat-eating habit unites us to primeval, ferocious beasts. Today's sophisticated party in an upscale restaurant, sitting around a table on which a pig's head or some exquisitely cooked fowl has been artfully disposed, is not essentially different from the tribe of savages crouching on the ashes around a cave's fire to gnaw at some bone of the hunted quarry. To the perspicacious gaze of those used to reflecting on what they see, the similarity will be obvious. The glimmering chandelier above, the immaculate white tablecloths, the waiters in tuxedos, the expensive silverware, the shiny Baccarat glass, the sumptuous draperies behind which musicians play chamber music—none of these trappings hides from the perceptive the stark fact that these men and women are here to devour the torn flesh of a dead animal and to gorge themselves with its entrails.

Considerations of this kind led many a philosopher to condemn the eating of flesh among human beings. Plutarch inveighed against this custom. Who was the first man, he asked (in *Moralia*, 993), who first decided to take an animal's cadaverous parts into his mouth? Probably someone pushed to this extreme by penury and hunger; someone who had already devoured the roots of plants, the bark of trees, and, desperate for food in order to survive, resorted to making use of the flesh of animals. But what excuse can be that of the men who lived in succeeding ages? Now the earth has been made plentiful; it is heavy with cultivated crops and bounteous harvests, and produces enough to support us. Yet an obscure form of frenzy continues to incite men to slaughter innocent, peaceful animals—for it is not on lions, panthers, or other ferocious beasts that they assuage their appetite, but on the peaceful sheep, the useful ox, or the tame fowl.

Plutarch, like others before him, argued that for humans to eat flesh is contrary to nature. And, to support the proposition that man is not naturally carnivorous, he cited the structure of the human body. If we had been designed to eat meat, he wrote, the gods would have provided us with the proper bodily tools. But we have neither a hooked beak, like rapacious birds; nor big fangs and sharp claws, like lions and tigers; nor powerful jaws and rough palates, like the bears of the forest or other meat-eating creatures. Instead our mouth is small, our lips are very sensitive, and our tongue is soft and supple. Then the philosopher extends the argument to the stomach. If men must boil and roast the meat before ingesting it, this is because otherwise their stomach would not digest it. By the use of condiments, sauces, and all manner of culinary techniques, men manage to deceive their palate and thus introduce into the stomach what normally would be rejected. For the stomach, like other digestive organs, is comparatively weak in the human species. It is an organ that can only produce "vital fluids too inert to digest meat."

In this assessment, Plutarch and his fellow philosophers went wrong. The fact is, the structure of the human stomach is much like that of carnivorous animals. Far from producing only fluids that are too inert, it manages to secrete acids so powerful that, given the chance, they could reduce the toughest metals to jellylike consistency. That our stomach can transform raw aliments and even foreign objects into semiliquid, absorbable matter never ceased to astonish the physiologists of yore. Some imagined that this organ accomplished its function by literally crushing, smashing, turning, pounding, and revolving the food. A colorful Scottish physician,

Archibald Pitcairn (1652–1713), thought so. He had read the writings of Giovanni Borelli (1608–1679), the Italian savant who applied his knowledge of physics and mathematics to explicate the muscular forces that move the body. Pitcairn took Borelli's calculation of the strength of the muscles of the thumb, extrapolated this information to the muscles of the stomach, which he had carefully weighed, and arrived at the astounding conclusion that the stomach was able to exert a compressing force of 400,000 pounds![7]

Others hypothesized that gastric digestion had to be realized through heat, and that the stomach was capable of generating cooking temperatures worthy of a bread-baking furnace. One knows not which absurdity is the silliest, whether to conceive of the stomach as a grinding mill, a cooking furnace, or, as still others maintained, a tank for fermentation. None of these foolish notions was based on systematic observation, and all would be corrected by the work of two exceptional men who favored the scientific method.

Réaumur and Spallanzani, or Gastric Physiology Unveiled

The egregious blunders produced by speculation joined to Olympian disdain of experimentation were avoided in the sagacious insights of two men whose names loom large in the history of biology and medicine: René-Antoine Ferchault de Réaumur (1683–1757) and Lazzaro Spallanzani (1729–1799). Both realized that gastric digestion had to be chiefly chemical.

Réaumur's formidable intelligence was exerted in a variety of fields, from metallurgy to entomology; in the former, his experiments redounded as much to the honor as to the economical benefit of his native France; in the latter, his six-volume treatise on the biology of insects became a milestone in the history of entomology. In 1752 Réaumur's attention turned to gastric digestion, which he studied in birds. Having established that the gizzard exerts an important triturating action, he noted that the stomach also produced a liquid with a potent solvent effect upon foodstuffs. He chose as his experimental animal a large species of kite common in France, because it has a membranous stomach that resembles the human stomach more than that of graminivorous birds. Taking advantage of the ability that the kite has to regurgitate what it ingests, the scientist introduced little tubes made of brass and filled with meat or other foods into the bird's stomach, then recovered them at different times thereafter. He observed that the foods were digested and could rule out a triturating action, against which the metallic walls of the tubes were effective protection. He was about to refine his studies, and no doubt would have carried them to a successful completion, but that tragic death visited him when he sustained a lethal fall while horse riding in the bucolic vicinity of his estate at Saint Julien-du-Terroux.

Abbot Lazzaro Spallanzani, from Reggio, Italy, was probably the best naturalist of the 18th century. He continued the experiments of Réaumur with unexampled tenacity. His concentration, assiduity, just discernment, and orderly method were altogether admirable. Like Réaumur, he started experimenting with kites, but soon expanded to owls, crows, and any animal that could yield the information he was seeking, not excluding mammals. A falcon fell to his hands. This presented some practical difficulties, but none that he could not contour. He tells us in his report:

A falcon was given me by my famous friend, abbot Bonaventura Corti, professor of physics at Reggio, and director of the College of the Nobility at Modena. This falcon was about the size of an ordinary hen [. . .] Soon I saw that I could not manipulate it as I did the other birds. His hooked beak and his pointed, acute talons did not permit me to force-open his mouth and to make him swallow my little tubes. But I found a way to make him swallow them without his realizing it: I cut the meat that I gave him in little pieces, and I hid the tubes inside some of these fragments. The hungry falcon hurried forth, took the pieces of meat and swallowed them whole. To make this deception succeed, it is necessary that the tubes be well hidden inside the meat; for, when the falcon perceived them, he took them in its talons, and tearing up the meat with his beak, he threw away the tubes and ate the meat next.[8]

It is a pleasure to read Spallanzani's original reports and to see the clarity with which he formulates the questions he sets out to investigate; the systematic approach to his researches; the ingenuity of the solutions he devises for problems encountered along the way; all of this told in a direct, concise, limpid prose, free, as befitted a scientist, from the rhetorical turgescence that still plagued the writings of many of his contemporaries, but at the same time marked by the sober, expressive elegance of a man who had benefited from a strong humanistic education.

He discovers that, under certain conditions, the gastric juice can digest the toughest materials, such as tendon, the tanned leather used to make shoes, and even bone. He wonders if it can digest teeth as well. To find out, he places two incisive teeth of a sheep within the brass tubes that he feeds to his falcon. After a stay of three days and seven hours inside the stomach, he finds that the teeth are eroded in those parts not covered by enamel. A new stay of four days in the stomach does not alter the results: the teeth's roots are completely digested, but the enamel-covered surface remains intact. His conclusion is appropriately guarded: falcon's gastric juice cannot digest the tooth's enamel, which seems to be a substance different from bone. As to tendons, he chooses the Achilles tendon of an ox and lets it dry several weeks until it hardens to the point that a sharp knife can hardly cut it. Still, the gastric juice of the falcon digests it entirely, whether introduced to the stomach uncovered or within the brass tubes.

Spallanzani realizes there is a great need to perform experiments with pure gastric juice applied to various materials under the controlled conditions of the laboratory. He manages to obtain some of this juice by the ingenious expedient of placing little sponges inside the tubes. After a sojourn in the stomach, the sponges are saturated with gastric juice, the characteristics of which he can then examine freely. By this means, he can study the digestion process outside of the stomach, in a laboratory flask, and demonstrates that outside or inside the organ, it is basically the same process. As his research expands, he scrutinizes the digestion process in dogs, cats, and eventually in human beings. After all, he is a humanist in the broadest acceptation of this word: a person who is intensely concerned with the welfare of man. The observations in cats and dogs, whose stomachs are similar to that of the human, had indicated that in man, too, the gastric digestion is primarily chemical, with a negligible contribution of mechanical trituration. Yet "this conclusion was made by analogy, and therefore was only probable." He wished for scientific certainty, but to reach this goal, he had to overcome new difficulties.

As often done in his time, Spallanzani experiments on himself. It is not without trepidation that he decides to swallow the brass tubes filled with various substances of animal and vegetable origin, to see what happens to them after their journey through the stomach and intestines. He is worried that a hard, metallic object may be detained in the course of its progress, for he has heard of cases of obstruction of the digestive tract that resulted in death. But he also reflects on everyday observations that seem to militate against that risk and feels encouraged to try the experiments on himself: "I could see that big seeds, like those of cherries, morello-cherries, prunes, and medlars, were swallowed with impunity by peasants and their children, and passed quite well through the anus without ever having caused the least discomfort." Soothed by these thoughts, the good abbot begins to swallow a series of bags made of cloth—the metallic tubes were at first deemed too dangerous—filled with diverse foods and materials whose fate after gastric digestion interested him specially.

His results are brilliant and unprecedented. Still, he has reasons to slow down on his self-experimentation:

> My stomach is not better than any other one; far from that, I am unhappy knowing that it is weak, as is that of most men of letters, and this weakness I feel in the slowness of digestion, which forces me to abandon my work five or six hours after dinner, even though this one is frugal, as well as by the indigestions that are caused in me when I take an amount of food greater than ordinary . . .[9]

To perform crucial experiments relevant to human gastric digestion, he had to have the means to acquire a sufficient quantity of gastric juice. This was problematic:

First, I thought to acquire that which human cadavers could supply, and I tried to get it; but soon I realized that the gastric juice collected in this manner was so admixed with foreign matters, that it could not serve me, since I wanted to have it pure. The little sponges placed inside tubes, which had been so helpful to me with other animals, could not be sufficient; I could only swallow two tubes at the same time, a greater number would have been dangerous, but the juice produced by these two little sponges was too scanty to be helpful, and the juice itself would have been mixed with other substances during its passage through the intestines. I was left with only one option, to draw gastric juice from my own stomach by inducing vomiting in the morning, while fasting; I preferred to irritate my throat with my two fingers, which made me vomit, instead of swallowing lukewarm water, which would have become blended with the gastric juice.

Twice I proceeded in this fashion and I obtained an amount of gastric juice sufficient to undertake some experiments, which I will describe. I wished to repeat this exercise, in order to obtain more of my gastric juice, but I had so painful a sensation, and such generalized convulsions, especially of my stomach, even several hours after vomiting, that my curiosity could not overcome my repugnance.[10]

As if smashed with a battering ram, a number of myths and erroneous notions crumbled under the research of Lazzaro Spallanzani. The whole extent of his work cannot be reviewed here. Suffice it to mention one example of the many widespread misconceptions that the abbot's patient labor helped to set right. It was believed that digestion was akin to putrefaction or that putrefaction had a large part in the digestive process. Thus, it was pointed out that the breath of lions, dogs, serpents, sharks, and other animals is fetid and disagreeable, especially after these animals are fed; that the aliment extracted from the stomach of certain animals is corrupted; and that the changes suffered by food in the stomach, even after partly digested, resemble putrefaction more than any other process, including the change accompanying disintegration by acids. Of course, the evidence adduced in support of these propositions was usually limited to the subjective impression that the odor and appearance of digested substances suggested the rotting state.

The meticulous observations of Spallanzani put all this nonsense to rest. By careful comparison of digestion and putrefaction under equal conditions of time, temperature, and other ambient circumstances, he showed not only that the two processes are fundamentally different, but that gastric digestion actually arrests putrefaction, which suggested that the gastric juice could have antiseptic properties. The latter idea led some physicians to apply the juice to ulcers and wounds. Gastric juice was also used in topical preparations, based on its supposed emollient properties (which it shared with other secretions also used in unguents during the 18th century, such as saliva and bile). Its use was also tried, as might have been expected, in dyspeptic states: the gastric juice of carnivores was deemed superior in this connection.[11] These measures were generally unsuccessful, and the state of knowledge at the time precluded a fruitful investigation of the alleged beneficial uses of human gastric juice.

Those two giants, Réaumur and Spallanzani, freed the study of gastric digestion from the many crankish notions, myths, and misconceptions that hampered its rational understanding. Thanks to those pioneers, future workers would be able to say, as in the colorful utterance attributed to the British obstetrician William Hunter (1718–1783): "Some physiologists will have it that the stomach is a mill, others that it is a fermenting vat, others, again, that it is a stew-pan; but, in my view of the matter, it is neither a mill, a fermenting vat, nor a stew-pan; but a stomach, gentlemen, a stomach."

One would think that, after the lucid demonstrations of those men, the scientific opinion worldwide bowed respectfully to the superior truth so conclusively revealed. Unfortunately, this was not so. Scientists are only human: they cling to their pet theories with uncommon obstinacy, as if the need to relinquish them were a personal affront and humiliation. Forty years after publication of Spallanzani's work, some authorities were still ready to swear on their professional honor that gastric digestion was mainly the result of the stomach's natural heat and mechanical action; the stomach as a mill and a stewpan was back in fashion. Reluctance to accept the evidence came in large part from the so-called vitalist philosophy. Vitalists were persuaded that living processes could never be totally explained in terms of physics and chemistry because there was "something" in life that was unique and beyond human comprehension. This "something" was called "vital principle," "vital force," "*élan vital*" (a term favored by the French philosopher Henri-Louis Bergson), or by other names, but regardless of the term used, it denoted a quality inseparable from living structures and impossible to reduce to scientific formulas.

Vitalists had long regarded gastric digestion with a feeling of awe. It was, they thought, unlike any other natural process. Raw foods of animal or vegetable origin are converted in the stomach into the semiliquid matter that they called chyme, and which they erroneously thought was always of the same composition regardless of the kind of food ingested. (Analytical chemistry was then in its infancy.) That two substances of completely different origin—animal and vegetable—could be converted into the same stuff during chymification was a source of their undisguised wonder; no known chemical process could accomplish that. Chyme was further processed in the intestine and absorbed into the blood. It then passed into the tissues, where it became an integral part of the living animal (hence the term *animalization*). It is not difficult to see that, from a vitalist perspective, it was difficult to accept that gastric juice could bring about the process of digestion in a test tube, apart from the living organ and independently of the vital force that informed all physiological activities.

In 1812 a prestigious French physician, Antoine-François Jenin de Montègre, reported to the French Institute a series of experiments presumably confuting those of Spallanzani. Like the illustrious Italian abbot, Montègre had used his own gastric juice in his investigations; apparently he had less discomfort in obtaining it, but it only served him to conclude that gastric juice had no significant role in digestion. (From the description of his protocols, modern commentators believe that what he probably collected from his stomach was simply swallowed saliva and some mucus.)

As late as 1825, a professor at Jefferson Medical College in Philadelphia quoted Montègre's work as proof that Spallanzani's conclusions were fallacious. The gastric juice theory, he said, was to be rejected on general principles, as it was inadmissible to propose that a chemical solution and the vital process of digestion could be the same. But even if it was shown that gastric juice had some solvent effect upon food, the professor went on to affirm, this effect could not possibly be the same as chymification, for the latter was possible only through the unique, vital action of the stomach. The length of opposition to the conclusive work of Réaumur and Spallanzani shows how difficult it is to rid the mind of personal bias, even—or particularly—among the learned. It also shows the pervasive influence of vitalism and its role in shaping the views of scientists in the 19th century.

Eventually even the most recalcitrant had to yield to superior arguments and incontrovertible evidence. But there remained many other intriguing aspects to clarify. What is the chemical composition of the gastric secretion? How does it operate the disintegration of foods? After the food bolus is swallowed, it reaches the stomach, yet it does not merely fall and sink into the gastric juice like a stone thrown into a lake. No, it enters slowly, and, as Spallanzani suspected, it seems to be grasped by the stomach muscles and directed by them to the exit orifice, the pylorus. The abbot of Reggio formed this impression from glimpses at the gastric movements of the few animals that he cut open in the course of his investigations. But these were very few instances, and he was the first to acknowledge that no firm conclusions concerning gastric motility could be derived from observations of agonizing or somehow benumbed animals subjected to the serious trauma of abdominal incision. Not to mention his often reiterated caveats that conclusions drawn from experiments on animals are not applicable to humans, and that reasoning by analogy is unscientific, misleading, and can never yield certainty.

Therefore it was necessary to perform extended observations on living animals—ideally, prolonged observations and carefully planned experiments on humans, but this seemed an unattainable dream at the time. General anesthesia began to be widely used toward the second half of the 19th century; X-ray methods that allow seeing the movements of the hollow viscera, not until the 20th. However, the unforeseen arrived. The accidental, the fortuitous, is something we can neither count on nor avoid; we may follow the threads that Fortune spins, perhaps even weave them, as Machiavelli pretended, but we cannot destroy them. Chance made it possible, in the absence of anesthesia or modern imaging facilities, to observe and manipulate a living, human stomach. Only this time, the concurrence of the serendipitous circumstances that brought this about took place in North America.

The North American Stomach Story

It is a story that has been told many times, but it brooks repeating because of its color, its drama, and its importance in the history of medicine. But also because it vividly exemplifies a kind of social rapport that is established all too often between men of unequal station in life. This is the relation between master and servant or commander and subordinate. One "looks down" upon the other, as is commonly said; the subservient man's position being lower, he must "look upward" to see his superior. From above, the vassal seems smaller to the master, whereas that one, gazing upward, magnifies his overlord. No one appreciates the other for what he really is. We might say that their optics are distorted, each one looking through opposite ends of the same telescope. On the other hand, it may be better to say that they do not see each other, but merely front one another, like two insentient stone statues placed face to face. For mutual regard and reciprocal feelings of esteem are possible only when in the presence of a certain sense of equality. This did not occur in the relationship that we are about to describe: one was disdainful, the other humble; and between the haughtiness of the one and the debasement of the other, no true solidarity ever formed. All that developed was a kind of inert complementarity, which is the very antithesis of active, living communication.

One of the main protagonists enters the scene as an ambitious, intelligent, self-assertive young American man; perhaps a bit swaggering and petulant, but these are attributes toward which we must not be overly critical, as they are obligatory concomitants to youth conscious of its powers. Soon he finds his childhood milieu in rural Connecticut too narrow a theater for his ambition. Refusing to settle on the "splendid" farm that his father had offered him next to his own, he leaves home with no more belongings than a horse, a wagon, $100 in his pocket, and we know not what golden dreams in his head. He is 21 years old.

Arrived at the little village of Champlain, New York, he becomes a schoolmaster, and this allows him to make a modest living; it also affords him the leisure to read books on medicine, a discipline that interests him greatly. Three years of this kind of life are enough, though; his restless character urges him on to seek new challenges. His savings stretch just enough to allow him to go to St. Albans, Vermont, in search of new ventures. There he finds the opportunity to become apprentice to a good physician, Benjamin Chandler. The second decade of the 19th century is about to start. At this time, a two-year apprenticeship with a reputable physician is all that is required to become a licensed member of the profession. Our young man is lucky to have a fine preceptor who teaches him those habits of systematic observation that make an expert diagnostician, and the attitudes and techniques of pastoral care that afford consolation to the suffering. Not much more was expected of the physician when the state of advancement of medicine could hardly raise any brighter expectations.

Thus, in 1812, young William Beaumont is a licensed physician. He is now Dr. William Beaumont, for such is his name. However, 1812 marks the beginning of the war against Great Britain. In September our newly licensed physician goes to Plattsburgh, New York, to enlist in the army, where he is appointed surgeon's mate and assigned to the Sixth Infantry Regiment.[12]

His desire for action and thrills is more than amply rewarded in the army. The pay is a mere $30 a month, but he is there chiefly for the excitement. Not unexpected of a man of his temperament and disposition, before long he clashes with an officer and challenges him to a duel. Luckily for the history of American physiological studies, the duel is refused. Then William Beaumont participates in numerous war engagements, vastly increasing his experience as a military surgeon. In 1813 he is with a charge against the British, who blow up an ammunition depot, causing numerous casualties. For two straight days he performs trephines and amputations, extracts bullets, sets fractures, and does what he can to alleviate the suffering of the injured. This intense exposure to trauma medicine would prove particularly helpful in his future.

In 1814 he resigns from the army and returns to Plattsburgh, where he meets his future wife, Deborah Green Platt. He enters private practice and in a few years begins to build a solid clientele. Yet this career is not without its troubles: twice, disgruntled patients sue him in the courts, and twice the feisty young doctor emerges victorious. Moreover, he has a friend in high places: Joseph Lowell, who has just been appointed surgeon general of the army. In 1820, as the restlessness of Dr. Beaumont begins to manifest itself again, his friend recommends him for a job in the Army Medical Corps. Now that the war is over, such a position has much to recommend it. He is appointed post surgeon at Fort Mackinac (Michilimackinac at the time), Michigan, where he revels in the beautiful and majestic northern woods. In 1821 he takes a short leave to marry Deborah.

For all its ruggedness as an outpost on the shores of Lake Huron, Fort Mackinac is no sleepy backwater settlement. Quite the contrary, it is the center of a very active fur trade promoted by the American Fur Company, which concentrates the commerce of this valuable merchandise from all the territories around Lakes Michigan, Huron, and Superior, all the way to the Mississippi country. In the warm season, the place is bustling with merchants, trappers, and the so-called voyageurs—men in charge of transporting trappers to and from distant Northwest sites, chiefly on boats, or *bateaux*, from French Canada. These are hardy outdoors fellows, inured to paddling and navigating rapids in their canoes, or, when the current is too dangerous, carrying their vessel on their shoulders along the banks. They also sail on barques filled with bales of furs. In any case, they face perils daily, and their lives in the wild are full of adventures, which they consign in legends and songs.

June 6, 1822, starts just like any other day of the busy season. Merchants looking for deals; travelers from various parts showing their wares; voyageurs who had come in their boats laden with the pelts collected over the winter; men, women, and children from the village, a few Indians and some soldiers from the fort. All these compose the motley crowd assembled around the American Fur Company store when suddenly a loud detonation is heard. Immediately, the word is out: there has been an accident, someone has been shot in the abdomen. Messengers run to get a doctor. Minutes later, William Beaumont elbows his way through the crowd to the wounded man's side.

The victim is a young French-Canadian voyageur.[13] His name is Alexis St. Martin. He is the other main protagonist of our story. He is lying on the floor in shock, intensely pale, his face covered by drops of cold sweat. The wound he has just sustained, due to a musket shot, is horrendous; those who timidly glance at it recoil in horror. This is not the reaction of Dr. Beaumont, though; not in vain he has seen many times the ghastly depredations that war can inflict on young human bodies. His attitude shows determination, every one of his movements is purposeful, and he keeps a cool temper that allows him to describe objectively the damage inflicted, in this fashion:

"The contents of the weapon, consisting of powder and duck-shot, entered his left side from a distance of not more than a yard off. The charge was directed obliquely frontward and inward, literally blowing off the integument and muscles for a space about the size of a man's hand, carrying away the anterior half of the 6th rib, frac-turing the 5th rib, lacerating the lower portion of the lowest lobe of the left lung, and perforating the diaphragm and the stomach. The whole mass of the discharge together with fragments of clothing were driven into the muscles and cavity of the chest [. . .] I saw him in twenty-five or thirty minutes after the accident occurred, and, on examination, found a portion of the lung, as large as a turkey's egg, protruding through the external wound, lacerated and burnt; and immediately below this, another protrusion, which on further ex-amination proved to be a portion of the stomach, lacerated through all its coats, and pouring out the food he had taken for his breakfast, through an orifice large enough to admit the forefinger."[14]

Not many people would be expected to survive an injury of this magnitude. "The man cannot live thirty-six hours," the physi-cian was heard to say when he first saw the unfortunate voyageur at the scene of the accident. Except that this time the victim is a brawny man, in the full vigor of his youth, used to a life of harsh-ness in the great northern outdoors, and endowed with a vitality that marvels his contemporaries. For 17 days, he struggles with what seems an impending death, stoically enduring the atrocious suffering of the gaping wound in his abdomen. All this time, any food that is given to him—and care is taken to feed him only broths and soft foods—comes out through the hole in his stomach. Careful bandaging, compresses, and straps have to be applied to avoid the oozing out of gastric contents and secretions. To sustain him, Dr. Beaumont feeds him, *per rectum*, what he calls "nutritious injections." He means enemas: the day of intravenous parenteral nutrition has not arrived yet.

Against all expectations, Alexis St. Martin hangs on to life. Not only does he survive the immediate shock and proximate effects of the trauma, but by five or six weeks, scar tissue is already growing. Firm adhesions of fibrous tissue have attached the stomach to the pleura and the injured muscles of the chest wall. As to the bullet hole, it shows no evidence of healing: it still opens to the outside. Surrounded by wrinkled cicatricial tissue, this orifice now resembles, "in all but a sphincter, the natural anus, with a slight prolapsus," in the words of Dr. Beaumont. This perforation measures close to 2 ½ inches in circumference, is located about 2 inches below the left nipple, and the total area of mortified tissues, now into a process of healing, is approximately 12 inches in diameter.

Whether the therapy administered by Dr. Beaumont—wine with diluted muriatic acid, and 30 or 40 drops of tincture of asafetida, three times a day—had any effect on the patient's recovery, or whether his natural strength and uncommon vitality are to be wholly credited with the outcome, is not for us to decide. The fact is that a year after the accident, all the injured parts were perfectly cicatrized, with the exception of the stomach perforation, which looked exactly as it did a few weeks after the wound was received. A fistula had formed communicating the gastric cavity to the outside. Unless compresses, bandages, and a tent devised by the physician were applied, the food and drinks taken by mouth continued to exude through the fistulous orifice. St. Martin could drink a quart of water and a bowl of soup; the next minute, if no precautions were taken, all of it would pour to the outside.

Now let us see what has happened after one more year elapsed and the patient has recovered his natural strength. To renew his former activities is out of the question. To embark in his canoe and venture into the northern rivers and lakes is imprudent, to say the least. He is illiterate, has no means of support, and the local authorities are thinking about sending him back home to his native village, north of Montreal, very far from Fort Mackinac. However, Dr. Beaumont hires him as an employee, to do chores around his house. These include chopping wood and other jobs that require some muscular effort, which the servant performs without apparent ill effects on his health.

It does not escape the shrewd physician that his patient is more than a medical curiosity: he represents a once-in-a-lifetime opportunity to look into the living stomach and to perform experiments that might throw light into many of the unresolved questions that still obscure the gastric function. True, since the 18th century, there were at least three recorded cases of individuals with gastric fistulas who were seen by physicians. One was cared for by an Irish physician, Dr. George Burrowes, who had no chance to perform any experiments, as the patient refused to submit to any manipulation and died before long. Another patient was cared for by the world-renowned Parisian physicians Nicolas Corvisart and Jean-Jacques Leroux, but they were altogether taken by the cares and concerns of the patient's management and did no more than a few desultory observations of mediocre interest to physiology. The same may be said about a third patient, seen in Austria by Dr. Jacob Helm.

William Beaumont is the kind of man who, once an enticing project has taken hold of his mind, will not rest until he completes it. Accordingly, in May 1825, he starts a series of experiments on Alexis St. Martin's stomach. These relate mainly to the chemical and mechanical aspects of digestion, salient concerns of his contemporaries. Here it must be recalled that he is not in the great capitals of Europe; he is not close, even in his own country, to any laboratory with a passable degree of technical sophistication. He has a constant supply of gastric juice from his experimental subject, but no chemistry laboratory to perform the needed analyses. Yet the gastric juice pours out abundantly, and it is no problem to collect it; that can be done without any distress to the patient. Once, it occurred to him to send a sample to a famous chemist in Sweden, but the transport took too long, and the sample was spoiled. Beaumont works in isolation, in Fort Mackinac, in the Michigan woods, and with no trained assistants. But he has an *idée fixe* and the dogged determination that would render him famous. With his rudimentary tools, he carries out literally hundreds of experiments.

Through his "stomach window," Beaumont observes with great interest the opening and closing of the sphincter placed at the junction between the esophagus and the stomach—part of "the mouth of the stomach"—that occurs during swallowing. He notes how it remains closed during digestion. He concludes that the volume of the stomach can increase without a concurrent increase in intragastric pressure. Everything that he sees, he records with prolixity. The doctor ascertains that the lower, or distal, part of the stomach works more vigorously than the upper, or proximal, part, and infers that it is in the latter where food storage occurs. Beaumont sees that fluids pass more rapidly out of the stomach and into the pylorus, and he watches the swallowed fluid coursing around the solid foods. At any hour of the day or night, he calls on Alexis St. Martin for a new experiment or a continuation of the old. Through the fistulous orifice, he introduces all kinds of foods and watches intently the effect they produce on the stomach. Having seen the difference in emptying time for solid and liquid meals, he liquefies the solid aliment and is able to determine that this hastens its passage through the stomach. This finding was confirmed 147 years later by researchers who used an electric blender to liquefy solid foods and observed the gastric transit with modern radiographic techniques.[15]

No doubt Alexis St. Martin is having second thoughts. He is not ungrateful and is fully conscious of his debt to the physician who nursed him back to health and provided the means of his sustenance. But to be reduced to the status of a human guinea pig is by no means easy to bear. The doctor, on his part, is relentless. Now he wishes to introduce pieces of bread into the experimental subject's stomach; now he pushes in vegetables, fish, or meat, cooked or uncooked, and sundry other edibles. After introducing the foodstuffs, he wishes to see what is happening inside the stomach, and he insists on repeating his inspections every so often during long hours, each time carefully jotting down what he sees. Or else he introduces the aliment tied to a string, so that he can withdraw it from the gastric cavity to follow the digestion process at various times, each time reintroducing it into the stomach. These maneuvers may cause discomfort to Alexis, especially when the doctor's scientific zeal makes him lose all sense of proportion, as when he introduced 16 raw oysters into the poor man's stomach.

In the remoteness of his rural post, the doctor has no sophisticated equipment for his experiments. But whatever tools he has, he exploits to the limit. He introduces a thermometer into his patient's stomach and records the temperature at various times and under different controlled circumstances. He notes that when he introduces a long tube, at first it encounters an obstacle at the pyloric region, which contracts firmly. Next this obstacle is relaxed, and the contractions of the pylorus impart a circular or spiral motion to the tube, "frequently revolving it completely over." Then it is suddenly drawn in at the pyloric extremity, so that when he lets go of the tube, it is "sucked in" to almost a whole 10 inches of its length. If he now tries to draw it back, it requires some strength to pull it out. The doctor's fingers experience "a sensation of a strong suction power," as in drawing the piston of a syringe against a moderate vacuum. Close to 150 years later, using modern imaging and recording techniques, researchers would be able to dissect the different phases of gastric motility associated with gastric digestion and confirm the observations made by William Beaumont under rather primitive conditions.

At length, the human guinea pig wearies of the way he is being treated. He is unable to verbalize his concerns. Too uneducated to articulate that he feels turned into a thing, nonetheless he senses, however obscurely, something deeply humiliating in the view that others form of his abnormal stomach condition and the uses to which his physician and benefactor puts him—to say nothing of the physical discomfort and inconvenience that his master's zeal for research sometimes causes him.

Truth to tell, this brilliant chapter in the history of medical knowledge shows a tenebrous side when viewed from the standpoint of human relationships and medical ethics. It seems to have been taken for granted that the value of Alexis St. Martin's existence was essentially reduced to serving as a display of the workings of the stomach. For one thing, no one ever thought of the possibility of treating his fistula. At least no one gave any consideration to the options that may have existed at the time, either to correct the defect or to alleviate any suffering produced by that pathology. All those with authority and medical knowledge who came in contact with him acted as if it was perfectly normal that he should exhibit himself to their curiosity, bow to their whims, and obey their orders unquestioningly; worse yet, that he should do all this with a feeling of humble gratitude for being able to contribute to the progress of science and the enlightenment of his betters.

Alexis St. Martin is a humble man, but he does not take kindly to humiliation. There is here a distinction of importance that occupied many a thinker, but which is often ignored in daily language. Saint Bernard of Clairvaux, the 12th-century Cistercian and physician, spoke of the difference between humility and humiliation—*humilitas et humilitatis*: one is a virtue, joyously and spontaneously assumed, whereas the other is coercive and provoked by others, who inflict on the subject insults, vexations, and opprobrium. Alexis remains admirable as a humble man when he humiliates himself willingly out of generosity and gratitude. He becomes abased and full of rancor as a humiliated man when he bows by necessity, against the grain, in hopes of a future benefit. For it is true that no one is ever really humiliated except by oneself.

There is a limit, though. The human guinea pig grows tired of seeing his dignity injured and his rights trampled on; and from his disgraceful situation, he draws a sort of ethical pride that impels him to resist more and more the impositions of his master. Unable to take it any longer, Alexis St. Martin leaves the homestead of Dr. William Beaumont in 1825 to return to his own village in Canada. The following years are characterized by Beaumont's irritated efforts to find him—which was not always easy—and bring him back. His efforts meet with Alexis's refusal, clothed in various excuses. The rustic man's letters, probably written by his parish priest, are humble and polite but unyielding. Their mutual association can no longer be the same. More than once, they come together, only to go their own ways amid feelings of frustration and disappointment.

Alexis St. Martin's reticence seems justified: the former trapper is now married and has two children. He cannot leave his family alone. If as a laborer he ekes out a subsistence living and is barely able to support them, without him they surely would starve. In 1828 Beaumont is assigned to Fort Crawford, in Prairie du Chien, Wisconsin. He succeeds in locating his experimental subject in Canada and forcefully bids him to return. Alexis yields and comes to join the doctor, this time with his family.

From December 1829 to March 1830, another series of experiments is done, by which a great variety of food samples is introduced into the stomach of a compliant Alexis. But soon it is plain that the same old disharmony is setting in. The irrepressible Dr. Beaumont is as peremptory and hard driven as always, and his patient as mortified and upset as before. There is no remedy. If, under the stress of being forced to act as a human guinea pig, the man is upset and protests loudly and vehemently, this attitude will only trigger new observations and perhaps new experiments. For is it not important to determine what may be the effect of these emotions on the digestive function of the stomach? Thus, for all reply to the angrily expressed grievances, the doctor sits down and writes that "fear, anger, or whatever depresses or disturbs the nervous system" has a noticeable effect on the gastric mucosa, which "becomes red and dry and at other times pale and moist, and loses its smooth and healthy appearance." In April 1831, Alexis St. Martin leaves again for Canada.

Once more, the fidgety and resolute doctor William Beaumont tries to make him return. It has been remarked that at all times the doctor dealt with his subject in a supercilious, domineering way. Although he had tended him assiduously after his accident, and later provided him with a *modus vivendi*, still it was never in doubt that the relationship was one between master and servant. When Alexis would leave the doctor to return to his native country, Beaumont did everything in his power to track him down and at times employed various intercessors to persuade him to come back. His correspondence with these persons shows that he was very far from ever considering the possibility of establishing a more democratic doctor-patient relationship with the man who made his researches possible. He asks one of these intercessors to visit Alexis, "if you can endure this disagreeable condescension," and tells another (Beaumont's cousin) to bring back the reluctant Alexis "dead or alive."[16] And to still another (his son, whom he entrusted in 1847 with the commission to go look for the stray servant), he writes:

> You will take him in charge as a private servant in traveling. Keep him in his place and strictly control his time and services. Allow no undue familiarity or suffer him to take the slightest advantage of your age and inexperience . . . If he should give you much trouble . . . discharge him at once . . . and proceed without him.[17]

Beaumont's envoys generally report to him that the man with a perforated stomach lives a life of harshness in wretched poverty, his five children walking about "destitute of clothing" and their father beginning to evince a rather inordinate taste for the bottle. Still, he is adamant about his desire to stay away from his job as human guinea pig. To Beaumont he answers that he recognizes his debt of gratitude toward him, but puts conditions on his return. These would be such as to ensure a decent living for his wife and children. Beaumont reminds him, in his usual imperious and reproachful tone, that his wife was very unhappy when she was obligated to stay with him during their sojourn in Wisconsin, and that it was at her tearful and unflagging insistence that he was forced to leave Prairie du Chien. Parenthetically, that Mrs. St. Martin's unhappiness may have had some justification is inferred from a remark by a fellow officer of Dr. Beaumont, who, passing through Prairie du Chien, had commented that "the place seemed worthy of its name" (the French *chien* meaning "dog").

After protracted negotiations, Beaumont offered Alexis a contract that was supposed to bind him to work exclusively for his
master, make himself available for the medical experiments, and
follow the doctor wherever he might go. This amounted to indentured servitude, if not arrant slavery, since St. Martin was selling himself to William Beaumont for $400 a year plus room and
board. Perhaps this was a measure designed to preclude the possibility that other researchers would appropriate for themselves the
precious commodity that the ex-voyageur—or, rather, his unique
digestive organ—represented. During the years when the doctor
lost all contact with him, and his intermediaries had trouble finding him in Canada, disquieting rumors came by to the effect that
Alexis flirted with other medical men vying for the privilege to
peek into his stomach. William Beaumont must have found this
intolerable: after all the work he had done and was about to publish, he would not suffer someone else stealing his glory. In 1832
Beaumont located his elusive patient and extracted his agreement
to come back once more.

They went together to Washington, D.C., where the physician, thanks to his connections, was able to enlist Alexis in the U.S.
Army as an orderly attached to the medical corps. Theoretically,
Alexis St. Martin was now doubly bound to pay fealty to William
Beaumont: as a servant-subject by the contract he had signed, and
as a member of the military by the obeisance owed to an officer of
superior rank. In reality, the enlistment of Alexis St. Martin in the
American armed forces was of little consequence: at that time, the
lines of command and obligations for orderlies were not as organized as they became later, and the enlistment remained without
any practical effects.

The year 1832 marked William Beaumont's last experiments on his increasingly unwilling subject. Profiting from a time when his master had gone on a trip to acquire medical textbooks and some equipment, Alexis St. Martin absconded, this time never to come back.

In the last year of his researches, Beaumont was able to recruit the help of only two prominent scientists among the many to whom he applied. These were Robley Dunglison, professor of medicine at the University of Virginia, who was originally from England and had come to America invited by Thomas Jefferson; and Benjamin Silliman, professor of physiology at Yale University. These reputable scientists, in particular Dunglison, made important suggestions about the questions that had to be asked and helped to plan the experiments fit to answer them. It was through them that Beaumont's work came to the attention of leading physiologists in Europe.

The following year, Dr. Beaumont published his historical book, *Experiments and Observations on the Gastric Juice and the Physiology of Digestion*. This work justly earned him a much desired fame. It detailed eight years of patiently accumulated observations that decisively ended once and for all long-held misconceptions about gastric physiology. He had wished to receive all the credit, and insensitively failed to acknowledge the magnitude of Dunglison's collaboration. Yet he was not happy with the reception that the book was given.[18]

Criticism came from vitalists who disapproved of his "reducing the stomach to a mere chemical laboratory." One of them declared the book "far too chemical to meet our approbation." Another one wrote ironically that the dissolving powers of the gastric juice were something like "the dream of alchymy [*sic*]." However, vitalism was eventually exposed as fallacious, while William Beaumont's researches were enshrined as a milestone in the history of medicine.

The book cost three dollars, which was high for the time. Dr. Beaumont was also disappointed by its lack of financial success. In 1834, impetuous as usual, he requested money from Congress. With incredible insensitivity, he asked Dunglison for a letter of support, which the scientist generously gave him. Some compensation was owed him, he said in his petition, for he had sacrificed his own resources out of compassionate humane feelings and love of science. He had taken into his home a poor, ignorant man who suffered a grievous abdominal injury. Since 1822, the year the man was hurt, he had fed him, lodged him, provided him with medical and surgical care, and cared for him, all at his personal expense; and during this time he, William Beaumont, had been able to perform studies that allowed him to make a significant contribution to science. Surely this self-abnegation and scientific achievement deserved the government's financial support? He figured that he had spent $4,000, but asked for only $3,148.75, a sum he arrived at by computing $1.25 a day for four years, plus various expenses.

In formulating his request, the feisty doctor conveniently forgot that the Michilimackinac County Commission had actually paid a woman for nursing services to Alexis and had disbursed some money to the physician as well for his medical services. Also disregarded was the fact that during half the time claimed as expenditure, the patient had been in his native Canadian village, under no one's care. Equally overlooked from the calculation was the modest pay that Alexis St. Martin had received for some time since December 1832 as an orderly in the U.S. Army. As to the significance of the research performed, there could be no argument: it was a major advance in the understanding of gastric physiology, and a triumph of American medical science. However, the United States at this time had no established granting institution for the support of scientific projects. There was as yet no organized process for channeling government funds to promote medical research. Furthermore, most congressmen were unaware of the true importance of Beaumont's work. His request was denied.

From then on, the life of William Beaumont becomes less likely to arrest notice. He was transferred to St. Louis, where he could continue doing research at the same time as practicing medicine. No longer could he experiment on Alexis, although to the last he continued trying vainly to contact him. Later, when his friend Lowell no longer had an influential post in the government, Beaumont was denied the facilities and the permission to extend his research in physiology. He then left the army and established a successful medical practice in St. Louis. His reputation was consolidated firmly, the value of his work was acknowledged worldwide, and in his final years, he occupied a prominent position within the St. Louis medical community. Coming out from visiting a patient during the winter of 1853, he slipped on icy steps, fell, and died shortly thereafter from complications. He was 68 years old. Beaumont was buried in the elegant Bellefontaine Cemetery; his funeral was as sumptuous, impressive, and ornate as was expected for a prestigious physician and famous scientist.

Alexis St. Martin survived his difficult benefactor by 17 years. He dragged along in a life of want. To one of Beaumont's many injunctions for him to return, he answered that he would certainly comply with his wishes as soon as some family affair was settled, but that for the time being he earned a living tilling the land and pulling heavy loads. This was probably an exaggeration, since by then he was in his seventies. Reputable scientists knew of his existence and would have loved to set their hands on him (or, rather, on his gastrocutaneous fistula), but that was the last thing that Alexis wanted. Still, some historians say that hunger and deprivation made him yield to the blandishments of a charlatan who paraded him from town to town showing his anatomical defect for a price. Apparently, this quack talked about visiting the capitals of Europe to dazzle the scientific community with his strange companion. A reputable scientist once interviewed Alexis and saw no evidence that he had ever set foot in Europe.

In the last stage of his life, Alexis St. Martin complained of not being able to tolerate the spiritous drinks that he liked perhaps too much. Indigestions came easily. The nature of his terminal illness is not known; he'd probably had enough of medical examinations, and expired quietly at home on June 24, 1880, surrounded by his close family, in the little town of St. Thomas de Joliette, 40 miles northeast of Montreal. He was 83 years of age.

Sir William Osler (1849–1919), internationally renowned physician who is sometimes called "the Father of Modern Medicine," knew of the studies that had been performed on Alexis St. Martin, and strongly advocated an autopsy. The state of that stomach was of no small interest for the profession. Alexis's wife and relatives did everything they could to respect the wishes of the deceased and to thwart those who planned to use his corpse for scientific purposes. They kept the cadaver for several days in a coffin at home. This was done on purpose: it was summer, and the body corrupted promptly in the warm temperature. This way they ensured that the tissues would be useless for any scientific purpose. Then the burial was done in an unmarked grave, so that it would be difficult for anyone outside of the deceased man's close relatives to find it. Lastly, the body was buried at a depth of eight feet instead of six, to deter grave robbers (known at the time to earn money by violating tombs and selling their macabre booty to anatomists) from perpetrating their execrable crime on the remains of Alexis St. Martin.

Humiliated and sometimes downright abused in life by the insensitive and privileged, he was again reviled posthumously by at least one member of that contemptible caste. In 1939 a curator at the University of Chicago, charged with organizing a donation of papers and documents of Dr. William Beaumont, came across some of his correspondence with Alexis St. Martin. In the margin of one of the letters that Alexis had written, the curator affixed his opinion that "the translated text of this letter is representation of many others by the surly, irresponsible, pecunious [*sic*], ungrateful ward and human guinea pig to his solicitous, merciful and generous benefactor." We can almost see the sanctimonious curator, his nose raised up in the air and looking down contemptuously as he deigns to address his invective against the whole lot of irresponsible, impecunious, and ungrateful unwashed who dare to refuse their bodies to science. All this said without a ruffle on his good conscience.

A more humane and enlightened stance was adopted by the Canadian Physiological Society 82 years after the death of Alexis St. Martin. Recognizing the invaluable nature of his passive yet fundamental contribution to science, the members of that learned group decided to honor his memory by unveiling a plaque in his honor. It was not easy to trace the whereabouts of his remains: it took some sleuth work from physiologists who visited his hometown of St. Thomas de Joliette. The funeral service had not taken place in the church, due to the advanced decomposition of the body. Therefore there were no acts or other church documents to indicate the place of burial. The grave was unmarked. Surviving members of the family were found and persuaded to allow the memorial ceremony to take place. They revealed the location of the burial site, which was in the back of the village church.

The ceremony took place on June 9, 1962. A tablet was placed upon which are inscribed the name, dates of birth and death of the honoree, and other biographical data. It ends with a simple phrase: "Through his affliction he served all humanity." Underneath, an exhortation that reads better in the original French, but which may be translated as follows:

You who read this inscription, offer, in remembrance of gratitude, a fervent prayer for Alexis St. Martin and for all the sick persons who, by submitting to the demands of scientific research, contributed to the relief of their brethren and the advancement of science.

Scatology

A FTER THE DIGESTIVE ORGANS have performed their respective tasks, what remains to be done but to expel the residue? Here, however, the describer hesitates; the writing stops; the narrative becomes difficult; every line must be carefully thought over and over. For the residue of digestion is repulsive, nasty, offensive, and disagreeable in the extreme. More than repellent, the unpleasant sensible features of excrement are profoundly alienating: they advert to death and corruption. Dead bodies undergo putrefaction, a process with disgusting manifestations that are overtly aggressive to our senses. Excrement, a daily sight, openly or unconsciously raises ideas of death, putrescence, and dissolution.

The organ charged with the accumulation and expulsion of digestive residue, the rectum, occupies the lowest position in the pelvis. The ancient Greeks, unconditional admirers of the reasoning faculty, established a hierarchy of bodily parts. The head, the seat of ratiocination, naturally occupied the loftiest station. In *Timaeus*, one of the last works written by Plato, we read that the head is separated from the thorax by an isthmus, the neck; and the thorax is separated from the belly by the diaphragm. This way, the noblest functions stand uncontaminated by the baser. In these partitions, the Greeks saw the confirmation of their ideas. Nature seemed to establish a clear divide between bodily functions and assign each one to a different level according to its relative importance. The head was uppermost, since art, science, and philosophy originate therefrom; and the pelvic organs are lowermost, since they are charged with the irrational, wild impulses of sex, and the disgusting elimination of excreta.

The Middle Ages inherited these notions, but, given the fundamentally earthy humor of this period, elaborated upon them lustily. In chapter IX of *Problems*, one of several works falsely attributed to Aristotle, a ponderous question is examined: Why is it that the expelling of wind in the form of farts or eructation is considered vulgar, whereas sneezing is not? Answer: because the first two come from the belly, whereas the latter comes from the head, which is venerated as sacred. Therefore, the wind of such provenance must be venerated as well.

The waste matter is not only disgusting, but also vile and impure. The medieval preoccupation with religion must have enhanced the tension between a heartfelt aspiration toward the divine, and the unavoidable, daily reminder during physiological excretion that the body is corruptible and must somehow contend with its own filth and impurity. In the monasteries, the monks had to get rid of all the natural excreta before the religious services. The 16th-century French satirist François Rabelais wrote with his inimitable, almost untranslatable, agile humor, that the good fathers, by an "ancient cabalistic institution," used to proceed in the following way on getting up for the morning prayers:

> They shat in the shitteries, pissed in the pisseries, spat in the spitteries, coughed tunefully in the cougheries, driveled in the drivelleries, so that they might bring nothing unclean to the divine service.[1]

The repugnant dejections were the Devil's due; for the Malignant One, the Enemy of the Human Race, hovers above all that is repellent and odious. This is why his hateful presence not uncommonly materializes when the medieval mystics visit the toilet. Martin Luther, in his *Table Talk*, recounts that the Devil appears to a monk in that very place and sarcastically asks him whether "a monk in the toilet should not recite the *prime*," the prayer for the first of the canonical hours, which the friars uttered at six o'clock in the morning (*Monachus super latrinam/Non debet orare primam?*). And the good father, imperturbable, answers him: "What climbs up [in other words, the words pronounced in prayer] is for God, and what falls downward is for you." (*Deo quod supra/Tibi quod cadit infra.*) More direct and unambiguous was the reply of Saint Bernard to the evil spirit on a similar occasion. Questioned by the Devil over the appropriateness of reciting the holy psalms while sitting on the toilet, the saint answered: "That which comes out of my mouth, I offer to God; but what I eject out of my belly, eat it!" (*Illud, quod ex ore exit, Deo offero; sed id, quod infra ex ventre ejicio, tu comedas.*)[2]

The saints were ambushed by the Malignant One while in the privy house, a moment of unique vulnerability. The military know that soldiers who withdraw to a solitary place to relieve themselves are no longer on their guard: while answering the call of nature, they are most easily made the target of sharpshooters or taken as prisoners. And how embarrassing a predicament! Medieval illustrators balked not at depicting the moment when archers chose as target the rotund, bare behind of an unwary foe that lowered his guard together with his breeches. To this day, a colloquial Mexican phrase, "to be taken like the tiger of Santa Julia," means to be surprised in the act of relieving oneself. The allusion is to a famous bandit of the early 20th century, Jesús Negrete, nicknamed "Tiger" (*El Tigre*) on account of his ferocity, who managed to evade the tightest police dragnets until he was caught in the Santa Julia neighborhood behind some cactuses, pants down, while egesting, and thus unable to use his weapon.

The terminal phase of the digestive process posed no few theological quandaries to medieval scholars. When Christ incarnated, and thereby became invested with humanity, did that mean that all the attributes of humankind, including those that reflect the misery of corporeality, became a part of the divine person? The Gnostics maintained that He "ate and drank, but did not defecate, [. . .] the foods did not corrupt inside His body, because there was absolutely no corruption." Christ said, "My flesh is food indeed and

My blood is drink indeed" (John 6:55), and "He who eats My flesh and drinks My blood abides in Me and I in him" (John 6:56). This ingestion by the faithful is supposed to take place in the sacrament of the Eucharist.

Now, suppose that, in a moment of distraction, the holy hosts are left unprotected, and a bold mouse—which until now has lived in some obscure hole of the temple—jumps upon the altar and, before it can be chased away by the priest, manages to nibble on them. Does that mean that the Holy Spirit abides in the mouse, and the mouse abides in the Holy Spirit? And without resorting to such a contrived situation, what can be the fate of the host taken by the faithful during Holy Communion? Can we suppose that the same transformations worked by the digestive process on ordinary foods will operate on it as well? Can we then assume that any residue, be it ever infinitesimally small molecules, will come out admixed with the feces and be flushed down the toilet? Incredible as it now seems, questions of this ilk tortured theologians for at least five centuries.

The fact is, our lowly excretion is not to be ignored. It is part of the world, it is part of our nature, and the most ethereal philosophies cannot completely disregard it. Thus, Chuang-tzu, the best writer among the great Taoist sages of China, opined that the Tao, "the Way," may be found even in human dejections. In chapter XXII of his complete works,[3] we read:

> Tong kuo-tse asked Chuang-tzu: "Where is this Tao [some translators write "God"] that you are always talking about?"
> "Everywhere," said Chuang-tzu.
> "You have to localize it," rejoined Tong kuo-tse.
> "In this ant," answered Chuang-tzu.

"Why so low?"
"In this blade of grass."
"How come so low?"
"In this tile."
"Lower yet?"
"In excrement," said Chuang-tzu.
Tong kuo-tse said no more.

This was a contemptuous answer of Chuang-tzu to his questioner, for the question being discussed was what the Tao is, and all the dull fellow thought of asking was *where* it is. But the sage makes his point forcibly: the Tao is found everywhere. Disgust is no valid grounds to deliberately ignore a part of reality, and a true philosophical system must be "all-inclusive, thorough, and universal—three terms that mean the same thing," hammers Chuang-tzu.

That the Chinese did not fail to give due consideration to this much-reviled physiological function in their vision of the world may be inferred from the fact that they had a divinity of the toilet. This was Zi-gu, "the violet lady." She was not entirely fictional but took her origin from a flesh-and-blood woman who lived about A.D. 689. To her misfortune, she was made the concubine of a high government official, Li-Jing. This man's legitimate wife, overcome by jealousy, killed Zi-gu in cold blood while she was visiting the toilet. Since then, her ghost has haunted the latrines, "a most inconvenient circumstance for anyone in a hurry," as an anonymous wit put it on the Internet.[4]

The Aztecs had their own goddess of the toilets, also a female, but in the grim, dark, and ferocious style proper to this warlike people. Her name was Tlazolteotl, and she was originally the goddess of carnal love. The Aztecs, for all their ferocity and warmongering, were prudes when it came to sexual relations. Female adultery, sodomy, incest, and abortion were punishable with death, sometimes by disembowelment. They transformed Tlazolteotl from the deity superintending wild, irrepressible, erotic passion, to a more sedate one presiding over parturition: she is represented with a child coming out of her pelvis, in the culmination of delivery, and covered with the skin of the sacrificed. They also gave her another name, Tlaelquani, or "eater of filth," because people told her their transgressions, and she forgave their sins. The parallel with confession and absolution in the Catholic ritual must have stunned the Spanish conquistadors, who rarely hesitated to adapt the ancestral customs of their vassals to the new faith they forced upon them.

The Aztecs assigned both positive and negative values to excrement. It was capable of bringing ills and misfortune, and associated with sin, but also powerful and beneficent, able to ward off disease, to subdue the enemy, and to transform sexual transgressions into something useful and healthy. Gold, the most precious metal in ancient Mexico (and eventually a major cause of the civilization's downfall, due to the greed it inspired in Europeans), was called "the sun's excrement." They believed that Tonatiuh, the sun, was a god who deposited in the earth his own waste as he passed through the underworld. Gold was eaten as a remedy for various diseases, just as desiccated, powdered human excrement was believed to be helpful in the treatment of eye diseases such as ectropion and glaucoma.[5]

Eating filth is assimilated to hearing the description of a sinner's faults. This association of ideas seems to arise naturally, since we find it both in the Aztecs and in Rabelais, who wrote that the monks everywhere are despised for that very reason, namely:

> . . . the frock and the hood attract opprobrium upon them, [they draw] the insults and curses of the whole world, just as the wind, as Cecias says, attracts the clouds. The undisputable reason of this state of affairs is that they eat the shit of the world, that is to say the sins, and insofar as they are shit-eaters they are rejected into their latrines, namely their monasteries and abbeys, away from public life, just as the latrines are separated from the house.[6]

The ancient Romans could not have been deficient in this respect: they had their own goddess of sewers and latrines. They named her Cloacina (derived from the Latin word *cloaca*, meaning sewer). The Latin word *cluere*, says Pliny the Elder, had the ancient meaning of "to purge" or "to cleanse" (*cluere enim antique purgare dicebant*).[7] The similarity of spelling with cloaca caused confusion; thus the name of the deity should be more properly Cluacina. The temple to Cluacina was near the Forum in ancient Rome, and on her feast day, all the latrines of the city were decorated with garlands.

The Holy Land was not exempt from latrine deities. To believe Rabbi Jarchi, a famous biblical interpreter of the 12th century, the Moabites and the Midianites, two tribes of the area, worshipped Belphegor, or Bel'peor, causing the Lord's displeasure (Numbers 25:1–9; Deuteronomy 4:3). The rites of this superstitious creed were celebrated on Mount Phegor, or Peor, beyond the Jordan River, and were full of shocking obscenities. Women votaries were prostitutes called *kedeschoth*, whom Saint Jerome compared to the priestesses of Priapus, the pagan god of fertility in the ancient world. Belphegor's worshippers were supposed to display all their bodily orifices in front of the deity, and, in Rabbi Jarchi's perhaps exaggerated account, bared their derriere toward the altar, relieved themselves, and offered their revolting, disgusting dejections to their deity.[8]

From all that precedes, it should be apparent that the excretion of solid refuse via the rectum is not the simple act that most of our contemporaries pass over hurriedly, name euphemistically, wish did not exist, and would forever ban from any decent conversation. Truly, it is an earnest act: a stern, implacable reminder of our corporeality and our finitude. In a way, defecation tells us that we are dust and shall return to dust. Hence the primarily negative way in which it has been viewed, with the exception already noted, much in spite of the baroque adornments that folklore and mythology have traced around it.

Human imagination, for all its portentous powers, has been impotent to countervail the strong association of malodorous, repellent waste and the idea of death and putrefaction-disintegration. But if we carry this repugnant, offensive waste in our bodies, would it not tend to make us sick? The desire to rid ourselves of the nefarious burden arises naturally. Here may lie the origin of a practice that dates back several millennia: the enema, or clyster. (Enema, from the Greek ἔνεμα and Latin *infundo*: to pour in; clyster, from the Greek κλυσήρ, from κλύζειν, to wash out.) This procedure has had an enormous place—still has, in many modern societies—in the popular therapy of common usage.

A hoary tradition supported by Galen, Pliny, and Plutarch, among other ancient authors, says that the Egyptians first implemented this practice. Legend says that they learned it from the ibis, a bird sacred to them, which uses its long beak to preen its feathers. The early Egyptians believed that, as the bird directed its beak posteriorly, it was giving itself an enema using the beak as a nozzle, and pretty soon they were imitating what they thought the sacred bird did to relieve itself of the burdensome excess. A Renaissance woodcut shows the ibis presumably engaged in just such an activity.

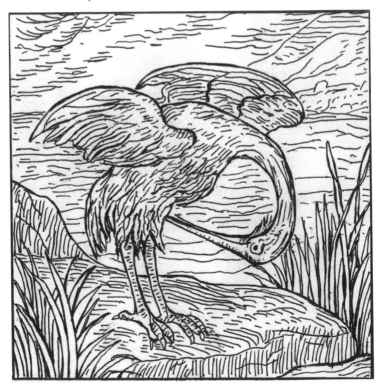

Fig. 2 Old engraving purportedly showing an ibis in the act of self-administering an enema with its beak.

Only the Egyptians, lacking a beak, had to resort to a reed stem for a cannula, and rinsed the rectum with the soothing current of the Nile. According to the Ebers papyrus, the world's oldest medical document, they were at it as far back as 1400 B.C.

At least two ancient Greek historians confirm the veracity of the antiquity, among the Egyptians, of the custom of taking enemas. Herodotus[9] says they did this three days of each month, in the belief that it was an effective way to keep healthy. Diodorus Siculus,[10] writing in the first century B.C., noted that the Egyptians believed that most of what is consumed as food is superfluous and potentially dangerous, and the best way to get rid of the harmful superfluity is by fasting and the reiterated use of emetics and enemas. That the ancient Egyptian civilization gave strong consideration to health issues cannot be doubted. It had a very large number of medical specialists, if this name can be given to practitioners of prescientific times. There were physicians who treated diseases of the eyes, others of the teeth, still others of bone, and the practice of many others was similarly specialized. Among them, some dealt exclusively with diseases of the anorectum. They were called *nero pchut* (some write *Nrw phw*), which some experts have translated as "guardian or shepherd of the anus."[11] These were the only health workers authorized to administer medicaments intrarectally. A German medical historian is quoted as saying that "in contrast to the popular contempt in which the anus is held today, it must have been an especially esteemed organ in ancient Egypt."[12]

The administration of enemas is practiced worldwide, but its reception was not uniform. Some human groups have looked upon it with unmitigated reproof. In Islam, views were divided: some swore they preferred death to injections in the rectum, but others viewed it with equanimity, deeming it a therapeutic measure like any other.

In certain African tribes, a calabash, or bottle gourd filled with water was the simple instrument for enema administration (when given to an infant, the fluid flowed through a perforation in the gourd's narrow neck, while the mother blew forcefully on a perforation previously drilled on the opposite, bulbous end). In India, the ancient enema syringe was made of the scrotum of a deer, ox, or goat and furnished with a tube of horn, bamboo, or ivory. The development of a syringe is considered a very important step in the evolution of this device through the ages. It is variously attributed to the great Spanish-Arab doctor Albucasis (full name Ab'ul-Qasim Khalaf Ibn Abbas) in the 10th century, or to a Marco Gatinaria, a native of Pavia in the 15th century.[13] The truth is that its development must have been gradual and cannot be confidently credited to any one person.

Thus, the history of the enema stretches from the remotest antiquity to the present era, and covered the whole world. But the "golden age of the clyster," so to speak, undoubtedly spanned the European 17th and 18th centuries. Here was achieved the Triumph of the Clyster, its veritable apotheosis. The procedure found a champion in a Dutch scientist who earned a place of distinction in the history of medicine. This was Regnier de Graaf (1641–1673), a native of Schoonhaven, Holland, who died at the young age of 32 yet having made very significant contributions to medical science. Among the most notable are a signal study of the function of the pancreas that preceded the work of the French scientist Claude Bernard by about two centuries, and a work that remains a classic to our day on the structure of the human ovary. Here, the ovarian follicles, known in his honor as Graafian follicles (small vesicles full of fluid and containing the ova—the reproductive female cells—surrounded by small follicular cells), were described for the first time.

Bred in the rigor and sobriety of a puritanical society, de Graaf was concerned with improving the method of administering an enema without offending the patient's modesty. The available devices that allowed self-administration had consisted until then of a receptacle or syringe attached to a curved tube, or cannula, so that the patient could carry out the procedure unassisted. But the curved tube that was inserted was rigid, made of wood, ivory, or metal, and the liquid enema could not be easily injected without moving the whole instrument at the same time. Such displacements jarred the tube in the rectum, causing traumas of varying severity, or allowed the injected liquid to escape at the side of the cannula. De Graaf designed new cannulas, perfectly fit for the anal orifice and provided with lateral orifices that minimized the leakage of fluid, and substituted a flexible tube of convenient length for the former rigid, curved tubes. This way, the new system became easily maneuverable, and traumas were virtually eliminated.

Like all innovators, Regnier de Graaf had to contend with detractors who found various false motives to impugn his work. Apothecaries, generally in charge of administering the enemas to patients, felt threatened with financial loss now that "it became easier for a man to give himself an enema." De Graaf noted, "The loss that may ensue as a result of administering fewer treatments is counterbalanced by the more frequent need of supplying the preparation required for the enema," since doctors would prescribe it more often, and patients, no longer afraid to show their posterior to strangers, would consent to taking the remedy more easily. Furthermore, he observed that apothecaries would be relieved from having to perform a chore that was filthy and exposed them to danger of contagion from infectious diseases.

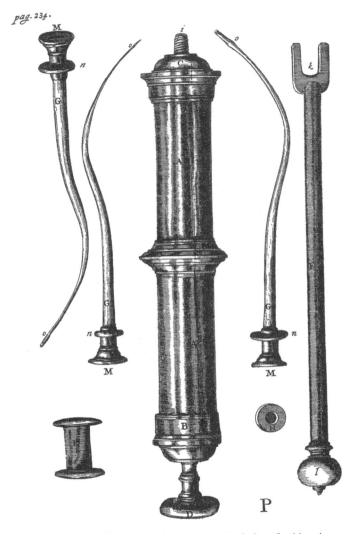

Fig. 3 Equipment for clyster administration, including flexible tubes, syringe, and cannulae, according to Regnier de Graaf (1641–1673).

De Graaf devoted a whole treatise, *De Clysteribus* (1668), to describe his thoughts and clinical experience with the enema.[14]

Perusing this work gives an idea of the vast place, to us astonishing, that clysters occupied in the standard medical therapy of those times. They were used to treat melancholy, to soften hardened matter in the bowel, to complement nutrition, and to introduce a number of medicaments. De Graaf recommended this therapy for the treatment of intestinal ailments, colic, tenesmus, diarrhea, parasitic infestations, ulcerations, and others.

Clysters could be "emollient, purgative, astringent, anodyne, detersive, divisive, or consolidating. Still others have received the name of nutritional." They could be simple or composite: the former, if they were formed of a single component, such as luke-warm water, mutton's broth, or milk; the latter, "if formed of diverse emollients, such as mallow, violet, marsh-mallow, wall-pellitory [plant of the genus *Parietaria*], [. . .] with which one makes a decoction in ordinary water, milk, or other emollient fluid. It is common to add, to this decoction, ordinary oil, or of violet or sweet almonds, or else butter."[14]

With increasing refinement and sophistication of the European aristocracy, the syringes themselves became objets d'art. There were some in finely decorated porcelain, others in gilded silver, ivory, mother-of-pearl, or gold, with esthetically carved adornments. Fashionable ladies displayed them among their toilette accessories, like precious objects, and rumor had it that Madame de Pompadour possessed an exquisitely fashioned syringe that could be seen in her elegant boudoir. These women, in the belief that clysters did much to preserve their freshness and to retard the ravages of time, became used to taking three or four enemas daily. Always ready to cater to the privileged class, a number of apothecaries promptly devised preparations of attractive colors and appealing fragrances, so that enemas came, like perfumes, redolent of orange blossom, lavender, lily, roses, and whatnot.

The reign of France's Louis XIV, the Sun King, marks the acme of the clyster's glory. Clearly, the ends of this therapy were subverted and the procedure was abused; it had been a medical procedure, but now became the fashionable thing to do. This kind of distortion is not uncommon in medicine; today we can quote many examples: Botox injections, psychotropic drug use, steroid consumption by athletes, and many others. Medicaments and procedures originally intended for specific medical ends are abusively deviated from their pristine aim, to be put at the service of lucre, vanity, or mindless fashion. In the *Memoirs of Saint-Simon* is consigned the well-known anecdote of a princess who, just before a theater representation at the palace of Versailles, and already in her dazzling evening clothes, received an enema in the presence of King Louis XIV. She stood with her back toward the hearth, talking to the monarch, while her maid, Nanon Balbien, placed behind her, held her skirts and administered the enema.

King Louis suspected that something was going on and asked what was the matter. At first, the princess hesitated and giggled. Upon the royal insistence, she said, "Do you really want to know? I am now taking an enema of water." "What!" exclaimed the king with surprise. "You are taking an enema here! How is that possible?" Upon which everyone burst out laughing. The lady's skirt fell, and the syringe, well covered and out of sight, was taken away by the maid. Women resorted to enemas to feel refreshed, to avoid headaches at crowded receptions, and for other reasons; men, in an age of gastronomic overindulgence, took enemas to prevent the untoward consequences of imprudently abundant repasts.

Madame de Maintenon, who became the consort of the Sun King at the end of his reign, was a prude. She found it offensive that people should talk about such matters. The mere mention of the word *clyster* she found hurtful to her pious ears. She used euphemisms instead, and for a while she enjoined the use of the word *lavement* (Spanish, *lavativa*; Italian, *lavativo*) which may be rendered as "washing" as an appropriate substitute. But this word too had problems. First, the acid satires of Molière turned it into a term of derision; one could not hear it without remembering the supremely funny scenes in which Monsieur de Pourceaugnac, in the play of that name, runs away followed by apothecaries who hold an enormous syringe in their hands; or the way the hypochondriac Argon, in *Le Malade Imaginaire*, is intimidated into taking an enema under the threat of being dismissed from the care of his physician (whom he did not need in the first place). Secondly, the Abbot Saint-Cyran, who at the time enjoyed the favor of the royal couple, protested that the term *lavement* was used in a Catholic religious rite, and that to apply it to an enema was next to sacrilegious. The sum of it all was that His Majesty ordered the members of the Academy to ban the said connotation of the word from the latest edition of the French dictionary. This they did, and for a while the politically correct euphemism at the royal court was *remedy*. Alas, even an absolute monarch has no authority over the sovereign power of words. *Lavement* had been let loose, and there was no way to contain it; shortly thereafter, it made its comeback in open defiance of the royal orders: *lavement* it was, all over again.

After the 18th century, the popularity of clysters abated somewhat, but throughout the world it continued in frequent use. Cases were known of criminal poisoning administered intrarectally; in the 19th century, there were advocates of dispensing anesthesia by this route, and some medications are still given to patients in this fashion. Today it is perhaps not used as indiscriminately or abused as often as in the past, but in many societies it remains a common modality of home therapy. It is common for households to keep the modern paraphernalia connected with its administration—no longer the ominous-looking syringes of the past or the artistically crafted ones to be displayed for swank, but the rubber bulb, or the rubber bottle, with the flexible tubes originally designed by de Graaf, albeit in newly developed synthetic materials.

As to the idea that to harbor a putrid, stinking material inside our body will hasten our own decay, this notion acquired some scientific respectability. That corruptibility and putrefaction signify death is a primeval idea; it seems to live eternally in the popular imagination and would not be easily expunged. Many a scientist must have been susceptible to this notion, but two men made it into the central preoccupation of their lives. One was a Russian, the other an Englishman. Their enduring impact in the history of medicine is sketched below.

Metchnikoff: Anti-Decay Ideologue, or the Colon Arraigned

Élie (in Russian, Ilya Ilich) Metchnikoff (1845–1916) was a Ukrainian-born biomedical researcher who shared the Nobel Prize in Physiology or Medicine with German immunologist

Paul Ehrlich in 1908. He was the youngest of five children born to a Russian officer of the imperial guard and his Jewish wife (née Nevakhowitch). It was this woman who raised him and imbued in him the love of study, for which he showed an early disposition, particularly in reference to the natural sciences. Metchnikoff grew up to be a biologist of merit; he became a professor of zoology and bacteriology at the University of Odessa.

He was 28 years old when he married his first wife, Ludmila Vassilievna Federovna, a woman of frail health. It is said that she was so weak that she had to be carried in a chair for the wedding. She suffered the illness of the century, tuberculosis. As the medical opinion uniformly recommended a benign climate and free air for patients affected with this disease, Metchnikoff took his wife to several cities along the Mediterranean coast, where he could work off and on, barely eking out a living. Thus, he found himself at various times in La Spezia, San Remo, Villefranche, Saint Vaast, Madeira, and other places.

His various sojourns on coastal sites allowed him to enhance his expertise in marine biology. This would prove immensely helpful to his later discoveries. However, his wife's health did not improve, and she died in 1873. Metchnikoff was devastated. He attempted suicide with an overdose of opium, but, fortunately, did not die. A few years later, he married for the second time. His new spouse, Olga Belokopitova, was well off. The newly acquired financial ease facilitated his stays on the Mediterranean.

It was while stationed in Messina, Italy, that he performed his seminal studies of phagocytosis in the starfish. He noted in starfish larvae, which are transparent, that carmine dye particles were engulfed by amoeba-like cells independent of the digestive system, which he called phagocytes; later he introduced small thorns from rose bushes, and these foreign bodies were also readily captured by the phagocytes. Similar experiments with the water flea confirmed his observations. This gave rise to what became a fundamental tenet of biomedical science: that the first line of defense against microorganisms that invade the body of man or animals, as occurs during bacterial infections, is made up of a class of cells uniquely adapted for the capture and destruction of such invaders. It is often asserted, with good reason, that this was the beginning of modern immunology. Today it is well known that leukocytes, or circulating white blood cells, are endowed with the ability to phagocytose particles, and that this function is essential for adequate bodily defense. The engulfing cells that Metchnikoff described are currently said to constitute a specialized system dispersed throughout the body, the mononuclear-phagocyte system, the study of whose biologic characteristics and role in disease is a crucial and complex part of the modern science of immunology.

Metchnikoff's second wife also died prematurely. Again, the scientist went into a depression; it was perhaps a Slavic melancholy that made him wish his own death. The story goes that he tried to commit suicide yet again, this time by exposing himself to material taken from a patient with relapsing fever (name given to infections caused by spirochetes of the genus *Borrelia* and transmitted by lice or ticks). Once again the attempt failed.

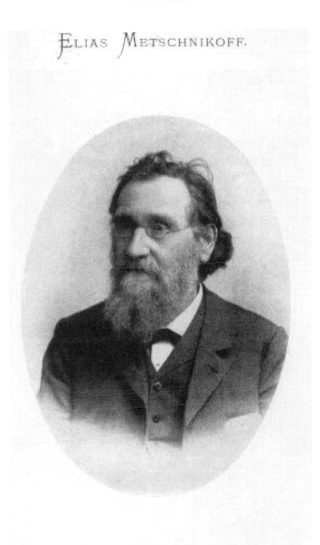

Fig. 4   Élie (Ilya Ilich) Metchnikoff (1845–1916).

He was offered a post at the Pasteur Institute in Paris, where he conducted a great deal of the work that earned him lasting fame. Metchnikoff demonstrated that syphilis could be transmitted to apes, thus facilitating the study of this disease, which until then had proved impenetrable. The photographs taken of him while in this renowned research center usually show him with long hair and untrimmed beard, not carefully tended as a fashion-conscious Parisian male might have styled it at the time. It is said that he commonly wore an old pair of clogs and always the same hat, on top of which he sat absentmindedly at times. His distinguished colleague Emile Roux described him as a "forty-three year-old man, who came out of the fringes of Europe, of inflamed face, shining eyes, entangled hair, and quite the air of a demon of science."

Metchnikoff held Leo Tolstoy, the great Russian novelist, in the highest esteem. He saw him as an inspiration, and throughout his life venerated the figure of the genial writer with undiminished, genuine admiration. Perhaps this reverence had something to do with the fact that he could identify with him. Both the scientist and the writer were Russians; both were ardent idealists; and both could be called votaries of what a learned critic once called "metaphysical extremism"—namely, the all-consuming preoccupation with the ultimate meaning of life and death, and the intimate conviction that they possessed the definitive answer to those immense, momentous interrogations. They met in 1909, but there is no detailed record of their conversation, which must have been fascinating. Both had grandiose ideas about the destiny of humankind; but the novelist, whose mystical temperament is well known, conceived

man's salvation through a spiritual reform and the faithful application of his own version of Christian principles; the scientist, on his
part, could not imagine the plenitude of human life divorced from
science (often the source of Tolstoy's distrust) and its attainments.

In the last decade of his life, Metchnikoff became convinced
that the rotting, disagreeable matter that we carry in our colon
is actually poisonous and accounts for our bodily decay. If only
we could be rid of the toxins that fill it, and hence infect us, our
lives would be much healthier and our longevity greatly increased.
He placed much store on ingesting lactic acid-producing bacteria
(*Bacillus acidophilus*) to prevent what he considered to be deleterious processes of putrefaction inside our colon. He wrote abundantly of the benefits of such ingestion.[15] Eventually, his advocacy
of the use of *Bacillus bulgaricus* therapy contributed in a very
important way to the rise of the yogurt industry. In our own time,
the study of the beneficial bacterial flora of the intestine, of which
lactobacilli form a most important segment, constitutes a field of
great consequence in clinical medicine, especially in gastroenterology and pediatrics.

In 1898, at the age of 53, Metchnikoff complained of tachy-
cardia, insomnia, urinary symptoms, and other manifestations
that, because of their lack of systematization, and considering
the labile emotional temper of the sufferer, may well have been
psychosomatic. Although reassured by his physicians, he became
very nervous and was seized by what he called "an ardent desire
to live."

Nothing is more difficult for a physician than the treatment
of an illustrious physician-patient with his own ideas about the

causation of disease. Believing that the fundamental cause of his troubles, and of senility in general, was a chronic poisoning due to intestinal microbes, Metchnikoff prescribed for himself a curative diet that consisted of avoiding raw foods (so as not to introduce more harmful microorganisms into the intestine) and taking large quantities of acid-forming bacteria in sour milk. As this regimen brought forth some relief, he started a veritable crusade to convince people that intestinal stasis and the consequent chronic poisoning by bacterial toxins were the true causes of many diseases and "of the too short duration of our life, which flickers out before having reached its goal."

As other sensitive spirits before him, Metchnikoff rebelled against the inevitable; he was pained at the idea that we must become old and die. These natural processes he deemed absurd; he thought of them as unwanted and unnatural impositions. Senility, like death, was what he called a "disharmony of our nature," and with singular logic, he maintained there was no natural propensity or instinct leading to it, for it is rare that anyone should wish to die, and no one wants to grow old. The truly natural tendency is for humans to eschew death, which is why, he contended—with less than objective evidence—children flee panic stricken from the sight of a cadaver.

Just as death and decay are the baneful physiologic "disharmonies" that we have inherited from our remote ancestors, Metchnikoff maintained that there are also negative structural features that are part of this bequest. Drawing support from Darwinian concepts of evolution, he proposed that certain parts of the body serve no useful purpose, and exist only as relics of a superannuated past. For instance, wisdom teeth are nothing but a reminder of our simian genealogy. The appendix is a useless structure, as shown by the perfectly normal existence of the innumerable individuals in whom it was surgically removed. "And the cecum itself, of which the appendix is only a portion," wrote our scientist in his book *The Nature of Man*, "is also degenerating in the human body," for it is very little developed in human beings (in comparison with herbivores, in which it is truly an organ of digestion). In fact, Metchnikoff thought little of the entire large intestine, "a useless and superfluous structure bequeathed to us by our ancestors." As in the case of the appendix, he pointed out, life goes on quite undisturbed after its removal. Indeed, long survival is possible without the colon, but the quality of life is certainly not "undisturbed."

Still, for all his hankering after immortality, or at least prolonged longevity, he aged like all common mortals and fell seriously ill as he entered his seventh decade. He told his friend Emile Roux, who came to visit him on his sickbed: "See how indissolubly my life is linked to the Pasteur Institute. Here I have worked for long years, and here I am being taken care of during my illness. To complete the bond, I would have to be incinerated in the great furnace where the dead experimental animals are burned, and my ashes kept in a flask in one of the armoires of the library." This, his last wish, was scrupulously respected.[16]

Metchnikoff died without appreciably lengthening his own life span. Yet his thoughts were not completely amiss, since it is true that the composition of the contents of the gastrointestinal tract has much to do with our general state of health. On the whole, however, he seems to have taken an unjustifiably jaundiced view of the human colon and its contents, convinced that man lives in a constant state of disharmony with nature, and that a colon is an organ perfectly useful for animals that live on a bulky plant diet but an aberration for those who, like us, feed primarily on quite another fare. More than that: according to Metchnikoff, the colon was not only disharmonious, it was plainly noxious, since it contains the innumerable bacteria that shorten our lives by producing toxic products. He strongly advocated counteracting the poisons he believed generated by the intestinal bacterial flora. Recalling the dietary habits of the centenarians he had seen in his native land, he thought that there was no better course of action than to recommend the consumption of lactobacilli-fermented milk.

Sir William Arbuthnot Lane: A Man of Action, or the Colon Condemned and Executed

A man obsessed by an idea, and shored up behind the solid ramparts of current scientific knowledge, is someone to be reckoned with. When, in addition to these qualities, he happens to be a surgeon, he is potentially a public menace; we must account him armed and dangerous. For a tribal lore—in force even today among health professionals—has it that the surgeon is "a doer rather than a thinker," whose salient attributes include manual dexterity, a knack for quick decisions, resoluteness, combativeness, independence, self-sufficiency, and a systematic distrust of tradition.[17] Commendable as these features undoubtedly are, they skirt perilously grave pitfalls: foolhardiness, scalpel-happy rashness, and unreliability.

This two-edged profile was the defining characteristic of William Arbuthnot Lane (1856–1943)—"Willie" to his relatives, students, and close friends. He was created a baronet in 1913 and since then decided to use his middle name, as more in keeping with his elevated dignity. (In the spirit of democracy, as well as brevity, we sometimes omit this middle name in what follows, and call him Dr. Lane.) He was an eminent surgeon who put his immense talent at the service of his ideas on autointoxication and in the process sacrificed countless healthy human colons. In a caustic satire, the humorist-physician Richard Gordon says that a boy with tonsillitis mistook the door of Dr. Arbuthnot Lane's office for that of the throat clinic, went in, and had his colon removed instead of his tonsils.[18] All humor aside, it is a fact that this renowned surgeon performed colectomies actuated by hypotheses that today are considered sheer fantasy and an aberration of medical science.

A historical perspective is needed to understand how one of the world's leading surgeons could have strayed into this wrong track. The idea that deleterious effects derive from the retained contents of the large intestine traces its roots, as we have noted, to the remotest antiquity. Most likely, it has to do with the intense revulsion that people experience toward feces. Yet it has been remarked that for this dislike to turn into a credible or pseudo-scientific notion, three factors are indispensable: a large group of patients who do not respond to the standard therapies of established medical practice; an environment characterized by rapid medical progress, wherein new diseases are being rapidly discovered and claims of new discoveries tend to be received trustingly; and a medical hypothesis that appeals to the medical establishment and resonates with the public.[19]

The first requirement has always existed; the third will occupy us later. The second requirement was abundantly fulfilled in the late 19th century. That was the golden era of bacteriology. An astounding number of diseases, until then mysterious, were shown to be caused by bacteria. Gonorrhea was causally linked to *Neisseria gonorrhoeae* in 1879; cholera, to *Vibrio cholerae* in 1883; typhoid fever, to *Salmonella typhi* in 1880; tuberculosis, to *Mycobacterium tuberculosis* in 1883; plague, to *Yersinia pestis* in 1892; a number of infectious diseases (erysipelas, throat infections, impetigo, and scarlet fever, to name just a few), to *Streptococcus group A* starting in 1881; diphtheria, to *Corynebacterium diphtheriae* around 1883 or 1884; tetanus, to *Clostridium tetani* in 1884; dysentery, to *Shigella shigae* in 1898.

The list is incomplete, but its impressive size in the short time it covers explains why the medical profession became partial to the idea that most, if not all, diseases were related to specific types of bacteria and their products, such as toxins, enzymes, and injurious proteins. Indeed, a facile assumption was that *all* bacteria were harmful. That a numerous and important bacterial flora exists in the organism to actually promote health was a notion that could hardly be expected to arise from contemplation of the havoc wrought by microorganisms in the human body, as medical researchers were showing time and again. Add to this the discovery that the intestine of the newly born is sterile, colonized only later by microorganisms coming from outside and taken in with food, and you will understand how the hypothesis that proposed a nefarious role for all intestinal bacteria was accepted so readily—more specifically, that the bacteria proliferating in human feces within the large intestine are the source of poisons that gradually enfeeble and sicken the body.

This climate of intellectual opinion prevailed when William Arbuthnot Lane was born at Fort George, Inverness, Scotland, on July 4, 1856, as the eldest son of a military surgeon. His childhood was remarkable in that he was obligated to change residence often: his father, being enlisted in the service of the British Empire, was subject to frequent reassignments. During the first 12 years of his life, Arbuthnot Lane attended schools in eight countries and four continents. He described his mother as "a woman of infinite courage," prompt to follow her husband to places where her comfort and security were not always ensured, and this while taking care of babies that came in rapid succession. The future surgeon was often lonely, his father away in military commissions, and he left in the care of military personnel. What this may have meant for his psychic development is for biographers to discuss.[20] By his own admission, the deepest marking experience he had was that of his years in Scotland, where he attended medical school.

Although in later years he had some troubles due to the fact that his Scottish medical studies were not recognized by the University of London or the Royal College of Surgeons, Arbuthnot Lane always spoke with fondness and heartfelt gratitude of his mentors in medical school. Much of his success he ascribed to the traditional Scottish virtues they inculcated in him: no-nonsense efficiency, practicality, avoidance of wastage, attention to detail, and a sense of thorny independence, together with unflinching adherence to the work ethic. The study of anatomy received inordinate attention in those days.

A contemporary physician summed up this approach well: "It was necessary to know the way round the body as the cabby did about London"—a solid grounding that served the surgeon well.

Arbuthnot Lane was 32 years old when, working at the Victoria Hospital for Sick Children in Chelsea, he developed a new surgical treatment for empyema (a collection of pus in the pleural space) which comprised the removal of ribs. Later he perfected a method for the surgical treatment of purulent mastoiditis (inflammation of a part of the temporal bone, arising usually as a complication of an infection of the middle ear), using gauges and other instruments of his own creation; these would not be the last tools he invented. Another great endeavor of his was the surgical correction of congenital cleft palate. But his reputation grew primarily from his contributions to orthopedic surgery.[21]

He was the first to treat bone fractures by open reduction and the application of metallic screws and plates, some of which he devised himself. This approach was anathema at the time, because it necessitated the transformation of a closed fracture into an open one, which was almost invariably followed by infection, which caused the death of nearly 50 percent of the patients who had the operation. Our man avoided this dreaded complication by adhering meticulously, fastidiously—with truly unrelenting rigidity—to the techniques of asepsis and disinfection, from which he never tolerated the slightest departure. So boldly revolutionary was his method to set fractures, that students were known to be automatically refused if they expounded on it while presenting the examinations for certification by official institutes and corporations of physicians and surgeons. Some student applicants were dismissed with the admonition that they should not present themselves again until they had discarded the dangerous, novel approach they had learned from Arbuthnot Lane, and could satisfactorily describe instead the conventional, accepted treatment.

Dr. Lane remained steadfast in the midst of all the criticism and opposition. A committee appointed by the British Medical Association conducted an investigation and ruled in his favor. His ideas prevailed, and he was vindicated. An anecdote of his life at this time reveals his character. Called as expert witness during a malpractice legal suit against a colleague, he was asked if the accused should have performed the operation whose disastrous consequences were the cause of the legal action against him. The great surgeon answered no, he should not have done what he did. The prosecutor then asked a further question:

"Would you have acted differently?"

To which Dr. Lane replied, "No, I would have done that same operation."

A bewildered attorney then insisted, "Excuse me, Dr. Lane, but didn't I just hear you say that the accused should not have done the operation?"

Impassive, our man rejoined: "You asked me if *he* should have done the operation, and I said no. But if you ask me what *I* would have done, I certainly would have performed the operation myself."

This pride was not unjustified. His colleagues' operative results were dismal because most had not yet become familiar with the exacting procedures that must be followed in and around the surgical suite in order to minimize the danger of infection; or else the surgeons were proficient, but their assistants were inadequately trained in this regard. It was not unusual in those days for a surgeon to rigidly enforce all the steps designed to stave off contamination, but then suddenly stop in the middle of the operation to scratch his head with a gloved hand or stick his hand in his pocket looking for some object; or an attendant might pick up an instrument that had accidentally fallen on the floor. Arbuthnot Lane, unyielding when it came to the procedures of antisepsis, and supremely deft with his surgical technique, was one of the few surgeons who could perform the open reduction of fractures and other similarly risky procedures, and everyone still expected the patient to survive without serious complications.

Some 20 years into his professional career, and his brilliant contributions having earned him a well-deserved fame, his attention turned to abdominal problems. The idea that the stagnant contents of the large bowel were the source of ill health was ubiquitous. Certainly it did not start with Dr. Lane. French pathologist Charles Jacques Bouchard (1837–1915), in his book *Leçons sur l'Auto-intoxication* (1887) (*Lectures on Auto-Intoxication in Disease*), had echoed Metchnikoff, coining the term "auto-intoxication" to denote this alleged chronic poisoning. In England, various medical authorities endorsed the concept that a sluggish bowel, by concentrating its contents, allowed diffusion of toxins into the organism. Thus, constipation was not a trivial problem: it was a serious disease in itself, as well as the cause of many extra-intestinal diseases.[22]

What sort of disease was this auto-intoxication that stemmed from a constipated bowel (or, in the technical jargon, intestinal stasis)? Since the toxins produced in the bowel allegedly entered the blood circulation and diffused all over the body, the manifestations could be systemic and multiform: urinary infections, arthritis, decreased resistance to infections in general, headaches, thyroid troubles, cardiac diseases, and even susceptibility to cancer. But a clinical description of a typical affected individual was still possible: the patient was usually a woman "of muddy complexion and with dark rings under her eyes."[23] She tended to be lean, because the direct effects of chronic auto-intoxication included loss of fat, wasting of muscles, and changes in the skin, which lost its texture and acquired an ashen pigmentation. Her perspiration was malodorous and her extremities felt cold. She complained of frequent headaches and tended to loss of control and melancholia. Because of flabbiness of the abdominal musculature, the abdominal wall gave way, and this provoked a downward displacement of the viscera. In the most severe cases, mental apathy turned to suicide or imbecility. The changes then became dramatic: the hair lost its color and could fall out, there was atrophy of the thyroid, and various organs could suffer serious damage, with the symptoms varying accordingly.

As with all diseases, important cultural determinants entered into the confection of so-called auto-intoxication or intestinal stasis (only 2 of approximately 60 names found in the literature for this condition). The Victorian age characteristically extolled certain values, such as order, temperance, respect of tradition, and an ultraconservative (some say hypocritical and prudish) concealment of the expressions of sexuality. Along with these attitudes, the cultivation of personal self-control and the correlative ability to command were virtues deemed essential in the men and women who possessed, and aspired to continue holding, the vast British Empire. In this context, intestinal stasis exacerbated the neuroticism of the Victorian age. For the bowel and its contents represent a threat to cleanliness, orderliness, and composure. A great anxiety was generated at the idea of "losing control" of the bowel, with its catastrophic, unthinkable consequence of either soiling, or its opposite, "stasis." Moreover, since injurious poisons were supposed to be generated in the bowel, this meant that people carried "an enemy within," and awareness of the danger hatching inside contributed to increase the neuroticism annexed to the idea of a sluggish bowel. Perhaps no greater ambivalence has ever existed toward the bowel than in Victorian England, where this organ was viewed with simultaneous skittish embarrassment and fascination, shame and fixed interest, shy modesty and hypnotic engrossment.

To exert "control" over the bowel meant to be able to empty it regularly, a hygienic measure to prevent the nefarious autointoxication. When this control was not imposed, overweening physicians did what they always do: blame the patient. This is an unfair alchemy that turns a sufferer into a morally deficient person; because undisciplined, the constipated patient was as contemptible as an alcoholic or a drug addict was deemed at the time. The physician became a stern moralizer. A patient unable to control his own bowel was "lazy, self-indulgent, unsystematic," and was equated to the idle rich, whose only purpose in life was to have "a good time," by which they meant overeating and overindulging in those bad habits that rendered them flabby, prone to sagging muscles and falling viscera.[24]

Arbuthnot Lane, who suffered from constipation himself, was wholly ensnared in the prejudice of the era. He came to believe that emptying the bowel once a day was not enough. It was a dangerous practice because it could lead to stagnation in the large bowel—the "cesspool" that had to be flushed of its contents regularly and systematically. He was generous taking laxatives and prescribing them to his patients. Later, having found that liquid paraffin was a "lubricant" with gentler properties, he took it himself, for he blamed his chronic constipation on the sedentariness of his occupation. He was delighted with the results, finding his sense of well-being remarkably improved. One of his American admirers, a surgeon named Leaman Bambridge, once gave a banquet in his honor. At the table, in front of each guest, was a little bottle containing liquid paraffin, ornately labeled *"Cordiale à la Lane,"* as if it were a fancy French liqueur. All the guests must have been converts to the idea that failing to flush the cesspool would bring forth the dire consequences of "chronic intestinal stasis" (a term coined by Lane).

Dr. Lane lucubrated on the pathophysiology of this condition with admirable imaginative flair (although, unfortunately, unburdened by the slightest trace of experimental evidence) as described next.

As the large bowel fills, it dilates and elongates. In consequence of the elongation, it tends to bend at the pelvis, forming a sharp loop that impedes the progress of the intestinal contents. As a reaction to this abnormal condition, the outer, or peritoneal, layer of the bowel wall forms adhesions, or "bands," that fix the bowel to the abdominal or pelvic walls. Soon blood vessels and lymphatics grow into these bands, which become better organized and more resistant, thus strengthening the obstacle to the contents of the bowel. The bands form veritable kinks in the intestine, rendering it incapable of propelling its contents.

Truth to tell, peritoneal bands are normal. Some are the normal suspensory ligaments of the bowel, others are congenital variants of the same, and still others may be acquired structures, perhaps due to minor inflammatory processes. But, in any case, they do not block the progress of intestinal contents, except extremely rare instances. This fact was not known at that time, for radiological and other techniques able to show that bands do not block intestinal movements did not yet exist.

Dr. Lane used at first conservative therapies. Later, misguided by his erroneous theorizing, his approach to the large bowel became, in the quip of a humorist, that of an angry, famished revolutionary toward the sausages in a butcher shop window.

Arbuthnot Lane met Metchnikoff, 11 years his senior, and was mesmerized by that messianic Russian "demon of science." The meeting between the surgeon and the laureate scientist must be called unfortunate, because its consequence was that Arbuthnot Lane's prejudice suddenly masqueraded to perfection as scientific respectability. All the uncritical opinions in vogue among the medical profession, and all the bowel-centered neuroticism of the Victorians, could now be clothed in scientific terminology. Evolutionary arguments were wielded in the most respectable scientific circles, where allusions to Metchnikoff's notion of a disharmony between man and his bowels were well received. A scientist could write with impunity:

Man has adopted a vertical attitude while his internal viscera are still arranged for a horizontal one. [In other words, the large intestine is a useless relic from the time when we walked on all fours.] . . . From his herbivorous ancestors he has inherited not only a bacteria-infested colon, but a tendency to a caecal diverticulum . . . The price to pay for the upright posture is to add another factor—gravity—to favor the stay of intestinal contents at the proximal end of the large gut.

The conclusion could not be blunter: "I am convinced that the large intestine is practically a useless encumbrance."[25]

Metchnikoff's writings developed the ideas that Arbuthnot Lane found so much to his liking. The surgeon was especially impressed by *La Vie Humaine*, Metchnikoff's opus with a Balzacian title. There the theory was put forward that to have a capacious large bowel is important for herbivorous animals because there must be abundant bacteria to digest cellulose. The large bowel is particularly well developed in mammals, due to the pressing conditions in which they spend their lives: they must always be ready for fight or flight. Given the existence of ferocious predators, the animals can stop to defecate only at the risk of their lives. They store the feces in the large bowel, which serves as a reservoir and therefore is functionally comparable to the urinary bladder. However, the conditions of human life are very different. Living in civilization, human beings are not constrained to lead a relentlessly active, fitful existence; nutriment comes easily and uninterrupted by the constant need to escape from predators. Creatures in which these conditions prevail, such as intestinal parasites, have no large bowel. In human beings, however, such an evolutionary adaptation has not occurred. Metchnikoff's implication seems clear: the large bowel is to man a "useless encumbrance."

Moreover, arguments drawn from comparative anatomy further devalued the disgraced colon: among birds, ostriches have a big large intestine and live only 35 years; parrots, in contrast, have a short large intestine and are the longest lived of avian species. The suggestion was not difficult to see: without a colon we would not only free ourselves from inner poisons, but we might live longer.

The third requirement for the creation of a pseudodisease, the emergence of an appealing hypothesis, was amply fulfilled. Strictly speaking, all this was mere speculation, and a little wild at that. There were no systematic, planned experiments to bolster such flights of fancy; yet in Lane's estimation, as in that of a very large segment of the medical community, they passed for respectable hypotheses. Arbuthnot Lane was ready to act upon them. Initially he made operations devised to bypass the large bowel. Later, when the clinical outcomes fell short of his expectations, his approach became more aggressive, and he performed total colectomies. A supremely skilled surgeon, he could complete this difficult operation in one hour or less time. Thanks to his fame and reputation, patients flocked to Dr. Lane from all over England and abroad. Out of his vast experience, he constructed a clinical typology of the patients he diagnosed with intestinal stasis, and he made the interesting remark that the women portrayed by the Pre-Raphaelite painters seemed to him to represent typical patients affected by this disease.[26] As is well known, the so-called Pre-Raphaelite Brotherhood of painters began in 1848 and drew its name from the admiration that its members professed for Italian painting of the 14th and 15th centuries, before the High Renaissance and in particular before Raphael. They had their own idealized way of depicting the eternal feminine, which they embodied in virgins, chaste medieval maidens, princesses, saints, and creatures of mythology rendered with striking realism.

Of course, each artist had his own personal way of capturing the spirit of womanhood, but in general they portrayed women of pale complexion, long neck, lustrous eyes, and a soulful gaze. Dr. Lane singled out three paintings with feminine figures that, in his opinion, reproduced the habitus of patients with sluggish bowels and auto-intoxication. These were *The Golden Stairs* and *King Cophetua and the Beggar Maid*, both by Sir Edward C. Burne-Jones (1833–1898), and *Nude Girl* by Gwen John (1876–1939). These two painters were members of the second generation of Pre-Raphaelites.

The Golden Stairs is an enigmatic oil painting that has caused endless debate among the experts. Eighteen young maidens (or are they spirits?—this is one of the points of contention) form a procession descending the steps of a pearly gold winding staircase that curves down the tall, narrow, rectangular canvas (it measures 2.7 meters long by 1.1 meter wide). Each one is carrying a musical instrument. They are clothed in long, white chiffon robes that come down to their feet yet allow us to see the gracile, slender bodies without any overt display of bodily forms. We do not know where these feminine figures are or where they are going; the staircase stops at the bottom of the canvas, after tracing a full half circle from top to bottom. There is no reference to any historical era; the eighteen maidens might as well be outside time. However, Burne-Jones used real females as models. For instance, the girl at the top of the stairs is his daughter Margaret; two society beauties, Mary Stuart Wortley and Laura Tennant, are two girls in the procession; and so on.

It is also difficult to see just why Dr. Lane chose these young ladies as representative of patients with intestinal stasis, unless it was their delicate, fragile air, their alabaster white skin, and the distant, ethereal quality of their appearance, which suggests a detachment from earthly concerns and the solicitations of the body. The good doctor had elaborated a clinical typology. He affirmed that, among his patients, those with dark hair tended to "loathe the sight of food, and frequently abhor sexual relations, while the red-haired subject rarely manifests these effects, even in the extreme conditions of intestinal stasis."[27]

King Cophetua and the Beggar Maid is one of the best-known and most often reproduced paintings by Burne-Jones. The critics saluted it not only as a fine painting but as "one of the greatest pictures ever painted by an Englishman." In it, the artist depicts a medieval legend, also the theme of a ballad by Alfred, Lord Tennyson (1809–1892), celebrated English poet of lyrical genius. King Cophetua, after roaming far and wide in his dominions in search of the perfect beauty, finds it in none other than a destitute girl. The painting captures the moment in which the king, entranced by the maid's ineffable beauty, sits at her feet absorbed in mute adoration. The girl's seat, on a higher plane, is much like a throne, for the scene depicts a reversal of roles: the ruler now pays homage to beauty, which is acknowledged as preeminent. The symbolism of renunciation of wealth and material values for the sake of the ideals of truth and beauty was much favored by artists and public alike in the late 19th century. The beggar maid has been called "the English Mona Lisa." Wrapped in symbolic beggarly rags, her pallor and delicacy are supposed to represent fragility, lofty concerns, and elevation of spirit. Was it not rather churlish, prosaic, and deplorable professional deformations that led a physician to see her as no more than a case of intestinal stasis?

The third painting mentioned, *Nude Girl* by Gwen John, definitely qualifies to pass as an illustration for a textbook of clinical medicine. The model was a young girl named Fennela Lovell. She was paid £15 to pose for this portrait, a considerable sum at the time. However, the relationship between artist and model was strained, for reasons that are not clear and which we may only imagine. Gwen John, the artist, was a woman who led a highly unconventional life. She was the lover of the famous French sculptor Auguste Rodin when she was in her late twenties and he in his sixties. Her brother, Augustus, was also a painter, who surpassed Gwen in success and popularity, at least in the early part of their respective careers. His life was as scandalous as his sister's, yet he wrote to a friend that "Gwen's passions for both men and women were outrageous and irrational."

Fennela, the model in *Nude Girl*, appears as a gawky adolescent of such a lean and scrawny torso that, conceivably, she could be diagnosed today as a case of anorexia nervosa. Her long neck emerges from ungainly, drooping shoulders whose slouch one may safely ascribe to muscle weakness. She is disrobed all the way to the pubis, where her left hand veils the genital area with what seems to be her blue dress lowered to midthigh. Her right upper limb drops stiff and pendulous along her right side, adding a note of awkwardness. A string collar with a small crucifix hangs between her small breasts. Contrary to the "soulful" gaze of the Pre-Raphaelite women of myth and legend, she looks half-defiant and half-distrustful straight at the portraitist; not a look of overt hostility or anger but certainly one that says "Let's get this over with!" She was so thin that when she was offered to Auguste Rodin as a model, the sculptor refused her, saying that she was too skinny.

If it were truly possible to make a presumptive diagnosis of intestinal troubles in any of the ladies in the three paintings mentioned by Dr. Arbuthnot Lane, it would be in this one. But there is reason to suspect that the diagnostic criteria that he used became rather lax, for he was persuaded that a very wide spectrum of pathology could be attributed to intestinal stasis, his main professional interest. Surgical excision of the colon was indicated, in his opinion and that of his followers, for patients who suffered from thyroid enlargement, gynecological ailments, degenerative conditions of the eye, imbecility, epileptic attacks, and skin conditions such as rosacea, acne, arthritis, and even baldness. "There is no limit to the number of diseases in which [intestinal] stasis affords the chief, if not the entire, factor in their causation," he affirmed.[28]

The fervent believer will see everywhere support for the truth and validity of his convictions. Arbuthnot Lane, already steeped in Metchnikoff's ideas and profoundly influenced by them, believed that additional support for his medical doctrine came from the work of other basic scientists. He saw the famous surgeon and physiologist Alexis Carrel (1873–1944) at the Rockefeller Institute of New York. Carrel, who won the Nobel Prize in 1912 for, among other things, his development of innovative methods of

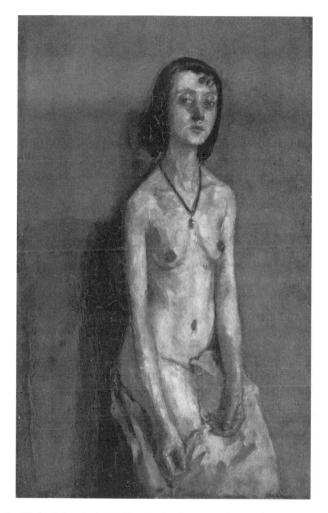

Fig. 5 *Nude Girl*, painting by Pre-Raphaelite artist Gwen John in 1909–1910. The young girl depicted was considered by the famous surgeon Sir Arbuthnot Lane as prototypical of the appearance of patients with so-called intestinal stasis.

vascular suture, achieved great renown promoting the technique of tissue culture. Uniquely adept at public relations, he caused a stir by extensively publicizing his ability to maintain living cells in culture for many years. Annual parties were held in the laboratory, at which birthday cakes were eaten to celebrate—in front of newspaper journalists and their photographers—one more anniversary of the survival of the in vitro cultured cells. The technique of tissue culture was new then, and Carrel skillfully flaunted the tantalizing promise of extended longevity, if not immortality, as a possible benefit of his research. Dr. Lane, obsessed with the importance of intestinal toxins in medicine, looked at Carrel's experiments, noted that the tissue culture media had to be frequently renewed, and concluded that this showed "the vital importance of the removal of the evacuations of the cells from contact with them."[29] In other words, the "evacuations" of cells reflected, at the scale of the cellular microcosm, the toxins engendered by the unevacuated intestine in the macrocosm of the human body.

The irony was that the work of Alexis Carrel was eventually discredited. His experiments allegedly showing indefinite survival of cells in culture were shown to be flawed. The cells could not be maintained alive as long as he claimed. The fallacy was exposed when, after many years, it was realized that the nutrient growth media was contaminated with embryonic cells (filtrates of mashed chick embryos were an ingredient) inadvertently introduced each time the medium was renewed.

As to Arbuthnot Lane's initially unopposed ideas, these too were now severely attacked. Which were the toxins in so-called alimentary toxemia? Skeptics pointed out that no one knew what they were or how were they produced. Nor did it escape the notice of sensible clinicians that infrequent evacuation of the bowel is perfectly consistent with good health and advanced old age. It was remarked that the intestinal contents are practically outside the body, since the lumen of the bowel is continuous with the outer environment. Nor could it be maintained that toxins were absorbed by a healthy intestinal mucosa, for there was no evidence in this regard, and some toxins taken by mouth, such as snake venom, caused no harm. Against those claiming that a deleterious process of putrefaction took place in the intestine, it was counterargued that the liver has a proven, great power to detoxify potentially harmful compounds originating there.

Advances in diagnostic instrumentation further contributed to confute Dr. Lane's hypotheses. For instance, as the use of contrast media made it possible to visualize visceral motility, radiologic studies of intestinal transit failed to show any patterns indicative of delay in patients diagnosed with intestinal stasis, and no pathologic abnormality was correlated with so-called bands and kinks. The claim that there was a latent infection ("subinfection") due to constant absorption of small amounts of bacteria from the colon could not be confirmed by advanced bacteriologic methods. Certain symptoms, such as headache and lassitude, had been thought to be very valuable in establishing a diagnosis of intestinal stasis or auto-intoxication, but it was shown that the identical manifestations could be reproduced by packing the rectum with inert material.[30] Removing the plugs made the symptoms disappear, thus showing that the latter were not due to the presence of toxins, as had been affirmed.

Starting in the 1920s, Arbuthnot Lane's concept of intestinal stasis and auto-intoxication gradually fell into disrepute. Other surgeons could not reproduce his results, and his own alleged therapeutic success did not stand close scrutiny and statistical analysis. He died in 1943 at the age of 87. In a hyperbolic panegyric, one of his biographers said that "those early observations on the mechanical effects of kinks producing intestinal stasis, autointoxication and abdominal pain were great gifts from Lane to medicine."[31] This high praise notwithstanding, the alleged role of intestinal bands and kinks is now relegated to complete oblivion, as is the whole conceptual edifice of intestinal stasis and auto-intoxication. No modern work of gastroenterology confers any relevance on these diagnoses. They are sometimes mentioned cursorily in introductory historic recapitulations of colonic surgery, but the commonest approach is to skip them altogether. This is not surprising: episodes of the history of medicine that make the profession look foolish are usually glossed over or ignored, and the story of intestinal stasis and its surgical treatment is too close to be dealt with equanimously. Perhaps this inattention is as it should be, since physicians must inspire confidence if their recommended treatments are to work optimally, and to seriously undermine our confidence in them is to cut back the efficacy of the cures we may need one day.

The truth is, Dr. Lane was no charlatan, and his contributions to surgery were many and of the first importance. Yet his career is held up by medical historians as an example of a genial surgeon who put his superior skills at the service of a faulty hypothesis, and in the process harmed patients by performing unnecessary surgery. Fanciful diagnoses and unnecessary surgical procedures are still being done today, but, as a wit put it with a kind of frightening, sanguine humor, "nobody knows which ones those are, until they are replaced by new ones."

The patients were not always innocent victims. Then, as now, many were active participants who, impelled by the collective neuroticism of the age, sundry cultural pressures, and their own personal conflicts, demanded that a surgical operation be done on them so as to rid themselves of their perceived evils. To the Victorians, one of the main demons to be exorcized was the "excrementitial view" of the world. Accumulation of filth in the rectum was a cause of dread and abhorrence. Nor should we feel complacent about it, for our times are still distressed by the same bugbear. The idea of intestinal auto-intoxication has been called "a medical leitmotif" that has persisted from remote antiquity to our day.[32] How powerful it still is among us is shown by the massive sales of laxatives and advertisements for these and other products designed to expeditiously empty the rectum of its repellent contents. This massive, universal business is supported by the idea, born in the deepest layers of our minds, that the excremental refuse emits noxious effluxes that deprive us of our strength and will ultimately shorten our lives.

Avatar of death and corruptibility, the rectum and its contents force us, better than any other organ, to look squarely in the face at our own mortal, corruptible nature. This part of our body seems to cleave mankind into two camps: those who would look the other way, wishing to persuade themselves that we are pure, disembodied spirits ever tending to soar on high, and those who dwell in our mortality, often with a morbid obsession for all that is material and putrescible in our being. Among the former are poets who sing odes to the perfection of woman's body, or painters who place her in the empyrean, amidst angelic and seraphic entities. Among the latter one finds mystics apt to agree with a saying ascribed to Odon, abbot of Cluny in the tenth century: "If men but saw what is beneath the skin, the sight of women would nauseate them. When we cannot bring ourselves to touch with our finger a spit, phlegm, or a trace of dung, how can we desire to embrace that bag of filth?"

Between these two extremes, it is better to think of the rectum as part of a wonderful, multifunctional, and still incompletely understood digestive tract, and its contents as nothing other than inert matter that is 75 percent unabsorbed water, plus short-chain fatty acids, cellulose, undigested fiber, bile pigments, and a marvelously varied bacterial flora by means of which we become an integral part of the ecosystem.

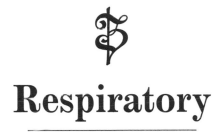

Respiratory

Like Leaves in the Wind

Among the many metaphors for the flimsiness of life, one of the best known is also the least accurate. The sword of Damocles alludes to the well-known anecdote in which a tyrant of ancient Syracuse was prevented from enjoying the pleasures of the table on account of a pointed sword dangling above his seat at the revelers' banquet, and suspended from a hair of a horse's tail. But a moment's reflection tells us that the danger in the story has been exaggerated: a horse's tail is a pretty sturdy thing. Its hairs are thick and made of keratin, a material whose tensile strength could ensure many an undisturbed dinner to the Syracusan—not to mention the fact that human nature cannot put up with indefinitely pro-tracted tension. We are so constructed that we simply cannot suf-fer high-strung nervousness for too long; the most ominous threat, if stubborn, will be forgotten; and Damocles, no doubt, got used to the dangling weapon to the point of thoroughly enjoying his postprandial liquor and after-dinner chatting.

Breath, however, is another matter. Insubstantial as it is, it can-not be forsaken. Stop breathing for one minute, and the anguish of impending death clutches you. Air is the life force itself: deny its entry to your body, and your life shall cease altogether. So it is that in the year 320 B.C., Diogenes of Sinope, the colorful founder of the Cynic school of philosophy, put an end to his life by voluntarily holding his breath. This, at least, is what Cercidas of Megalopolis said in his *Melambi*, satirical poems of lyrical tone:

No, of course not, the quondam Sinopean is no more.

The famous man of the staff and folded mantle, who lived out in the open,

Climbed up to heaven by pursing his lips against his teeth to hold his breath.

For he was truly Diogenes—the son of Zeus and heaven's dog.[1]

Of course, we find it hard to believe that anyone can escape from this life by voluntarily holding the breath, even though Diogenes was approaching his 90th birthday, an age when the stays of our existence are likely to be weakened, worn out, and most eas-ily toppled. Still more unbelievable, in my view, is the claim held by some that he strangled himself to death with his own hands.

But there is still another version: that the philosopher "was seized by a strong colic after having devoured a raw octopus." A less dignifying end for a man, no doubt, but more credible of a Greek, whose partiality for seafood must have extended to uncooked fare; especially so for a philosopher whose professed ideal was to live like a dog. On his grave, a column was raised, topped by a sculpture of a dog in the celebrated marble of Paros.

In any case, the end of Diogenes the Cynic must have been impressive. Breath-holding spells always are. Patients repeatedly subject to such crises, as in a rare complication following Parkinson's disease or encephalitis, stop breathing during inspiration. The face rapidly acquires a bluish tinge; the muscles of the chest contract, as in a spasm; the muscles of the neck do likewise; the veins of the face and neck become engorged; the bloodshot eyes seem to protrude from the orbits; the bluishness of the skin quickly deepens; the whole *facies* seems to reflect a desperate, anguished attempt to overcome an obstacle that impedes respiration; and these manifestations may be accompanied, in postencephalitic patients, by bizarre movements, facial distortion, contractures of limb and back muscles, and sometimes loss of consciousness.[2] The whole episode does not last much more than a minute, but to the sufferer and the witnesses, it seems an eternity.

Poets and philosophers, when adverting to the fragility of our lives, never came up with a better metaphor than one that seems crafted by physiologists: *life is breath*. None more graphic or more truthful: fleeting, like a whiff; insubstantial, like air itself. Which is why the connection between life and breath became anchored in language. The Greek word *psyche*, like the Latin word *anima*, alluded to breath as well as air, and in time both came to refer to the soul. Life—as this word was understood for ages—enters into us as we take in our first breath and leaves us when, as the common expression puts it, we "breathe our last."

Hence the unbearable anguish, desperation, and urgency that seize all who witness the sudden, unanticipated stoppage of breathing in a human being. A more grievous spectacle can scarcely be imagined, especially when the victim's age and circumstances did not portend such a cruel event. It seems natural to try to do anything to revive the person so stricken; almost instinctive to attempt to restore the lost breath by blowing into the arrested lungs the precious air that keeps life going. Still, medical historians generally concur in dating the first documented instance of such a procedure as late as the 18th century. It was performed on an adult man by a Scottish surgeon, William Tossach.

It happened on December 3, 1732, at Alloa, Scotland. A coal-pit miner named James Blair fell from a coal mine's stairs. His coworkers brought him out after he had been lying unconscious in the pit for about three-quarters of an hour. The surgeon found him pulseless, covered with coal dust, his eyes and mouth wide open, immobile, limp, having no detectable heartbeat, and manifesting the grim coldness of death. In the then current state of medical knowledge, he could be said to be, for all practical purposes, dead. Then William Tossach, impelled perhaps by anguish and desperation, applied his mouth against the miner's and blew his breath as strongly as he could. But, he tells us in his written report published 12 years later (those were the days, still blessedly ignorant of "publish or perish"!), as he "forgot to stop his Nostrils, all the Air came out at them. Wherefore taking hold of them with one hand and holding my other on his breast . . . I blew again my breath as strong as I could, raising his Chest fully with it; and immediately I felt six or seven very quick Beats of the heart; his Thorax continued to play, and the Pulse was felt soon after in the Arteries."[3]

Next he did what every self-respecting medico would have done at the time: he opened a vein of his patient and bled him copiously. At first, for about a quarter hour, the blood would come out in drops only (since the man was still in shock), but afterward it ran freely. Proof of the benefit of Tossach's ministrations was that after less than one hour of unconsciousness, during which the miner's lungs "continued to play" after the physician had "set them in Motion," the man began to yawn, then to move his eyelids (his eyes and mouth had remained open all the time of his unconsciousness), then to move his hands and feet, and in one more hour he came back to his senses and was able to drink, although he remembered nothing that had happened since the time of his fall into the pit.

Although acknowledged as the "founding moment" of the therapeutic procedure of mouth-to-mouth respiration, this episode had many predecessors, some of which go back to biblical times. Historians often refer to the Old Testament's passage in which Elisha revives the Shunammite child:

And he went up and lay upon the child, and put his mouth upon his mouth, and his eyes upon his eyes, and his hands upon his hands: and he stretched himself upon the child; and the flesh of the child waxed warm.

Then he returned, and walked in the house to and fro: and went up and stretched himself upon him: and the

child sneezed seven times, and the child opened his eyes
(2 Kings 4:34–35).

The passage is certainly allusive to a dramatic intervention and
a therapeutic success, although there is no mention of Elisha actually blowing into the child's airway. Yet these biblical verses will
continue to be quoted in connection with the history of resuscita-
tive maneuvers, if only for their vivid depiction of what must have
been a startling occurrence.

The narrative was bound to capture the attention of artists.
Lord Frederick Leighton (1830–1896), the academic Victorian
English painter, left an impressive depiction of the scene. One
wonders if Lord Leighton, as the son and grandson of prominent
physicians, was especially sensitive to a spectacle of man's efforts
to wrest a life from the very jaws of death. With strong contrast of
light and shades, which cannot fail to evoke Caravaggio's drama-
tism, Leighton bodied forth still another contrasting drama,
thus reduplicating the tension experienced by the viewer: an old,
bearded, bald, and portly Elisha, bends to juxtapose his withered
features to the juvenile radiance of an exanimate, pale, angelic child.
A moment later, we know, he will put "his mouth upon his mouth
and his eyes upon his eyes and his hand upon his hands." And not
much later, the child will have recovered his senses.

After the moment captured by Leighton's artistry, things re-
verted to what they were meant to be: the youth's spirit, plentiful
and effervescent, and Elisha's, dull and rare; the boy's pulse strong
and quick, Elisha's, weak and slow. But this return to preappointed
conditions, was it the work of a miracle or just a physiologic
change? Medical historians are divided. Some think that merely

by warming his body, Elisha may have brought the child out of a comatose state, either from sunstroke or from a minor cerebral bleeding.[4] Others believe that he was performing one more miracle and insist that there is no record of his having actually blown into the child's mouth.[5, 6] Nor was his curative method unique. Elisha's predecessor, Elijah, raised the apparently dead son of the widow of Zarephath by proceeding in a very similar manner: he "stretched himself upon the child three times, and cried unto the Lord, and said, O Lord, my God, I pray thee, let this child's soul come into him again" (1 Kings 17: 21).

Failure to take in the first breath carries a unique poignancy. The fateful scene most often takes place in the delivery suite of a hospital. A new human being has just emerged from the mother's womb: the spectacle is supposed to be an occasion for rejoicing and celebration. But, lo! the child lies limp, silent, and ominously immobile on the table. The burgeoning life is dangerously close to extinction. With no effort to utter a cry or to draw in the slightest whiff of air, that baby looks like the very emblem of premature death: ruin before its time, decay before maturity—passage from the nothingness preceding existence to the nothingness of terminal dissolution, without so much as that fleeting interval of light and warmth that we call life. Seconds pass that seem eternities, and each one increases tenfold the observers' anxiety. For it is plain that with every second, the chances for recovery diminish. As the newly born turns blue, an imperious inner voice seems to cry: "The child is dying! Oh God, let's bring him back! Let's bring him back! Let's do something!"

No doubt it was obeying this urgent call that the ancient midwives decided to blow their own breath into an asphyxiating baby's lungs. Elisha and Elijah's claims for primacy as discoverers of the method of mouth-to-mouth rescue breathing may be debatable, but it seems certain that Hebrew midwives were putting it into practice since biblical times. At least, there is a tradition, preserved in such writings as the Babylonian Talmud, *Midrash Rabbah* (of the 11th and 12th centuries), and others, to the effect that midwives assisted the newly born by blowing into their nostrils.[7] From these sources, it may be inferred that this is what Puah, a midwife mentioned by name in the Old Testament (Exodus 1:15–17), did to protect the Jewish newborn babies from the ill-advised rigors of the Egyptian pharaoh.

To promote the initiation of breathing is an enormous responsibility. How much greater when it was the life of newborn princes that fell into the hands of midwives. From the diary kept by a remarkable 16th-century French midwife, Louise Bourgeois, we are informed of the incidents attending the birth of Louis XIII, the successor of King Henri IV of France.

Apparently, the infant's state was precarious, in consequence of a very difficult, prolonged parturition. Louise Bourgeois receives him into the soft, carefully prepared sheets and covers, and wraps him very well, but she is worried by his looks. He seems prey to a marked "weakness" (this term included a variety of neonatal complications, including prematurity), and draws breath feebly, infrequently, and irregularly. The reigning monarch approaches, looks at the baby's face and turns, consternated, toward the midwife. This one, admirably preserving her cool temper, sees that the king is worried, but, remaining much in command of the situation, asks one of the royal valets de chambre, a Monsieur de Lozeray, to bring a bottle of wine.

He brings a bottle, and she asks for a spoon, and while the king is holding the bottle, she says to him, "Sire, if it were any other infant, I would put wine in my mouth, and would give it to him, for fear that the weakness might last too long." The king, immediately pressing the bottle against her mouth, answers, "Do as you would do to any other [child]." Louise Bourgeois writes: "I filled my mouth with wine, and I blew it into his; and at the very same time he came back to his senses, and relished the wine which I had given him."[8]

Louis XIII the infant must have responded to the midwife's breath, a rudimentary form of artificial ventilation. That it came with a good dose of spirits must perhaps be deemed a national quirk. Considering that the place was France, and the wine from the royal caves, it must not have been from an inferior vintage; and who is to say that ingress into this vale of tears is not better for being fostered by the double buoyancy of air and good wine? Until the properly controlled study is done, the better part of prudence is to subscribe to the American popular wisdom that decrees "different strokes for different folks"—although perhaps in this case it is more appropriate to say, "Chacun à son goût" ("To each his own taste").

It is not surprising that midwives knew what to do in such dire emergencies. They had learned their art from a rich experience accumulated through the centuries, whereas medical doctors (all of them male at the time) were kept away from attending births; this task fell entirely to women until well into the Enlightenment. Learned doctors who spoke Latin and wore imposing robes would not soil themselves with the blood and excretions of parturient women. Thus, even when physicians had heard of this practice or witnessed its performance, their ideas remained pitifully confused. In 1472 Paul Bagellardus, professor at Padua and author of the first known textbook of pediatrics, wrote that if the midwife should find a suffering newborn, presumably in the throes of asphyxia but "warm, not black, she should blow into its mouth if it has no respiration." (*Si reperiret ipsu calidu no nigru deber inflare in os eius ipso no habete respiratione.*)[9] Sound advice, no doubt, which according to a commentator was immediately ruined by the phrase that followed: "or into its anus" (*aut in anu eius*). The author leaves the reader wondering how on earth this could be accomplished!

It is astonishing to remark how utterly erratic and misconceived was the theoretical basis of respiratory medicine. Only by supposing it mired in the most bizarre speculations can we account for some therapeutic measures used to combat asphyxiation, as in drowning. Well into the Age of Enlightenment, a published method to obtain the recovery of persons seemingly drowned recommended, first, to strip them of their clothes, rub them vigorously, place them in a warm place near the fire or wrap them well in blankets, give them mouth-to-mouth respiration, and then "introduce the small end of a lighted tobacco pipe into the fundament, putting a paper pricked full of holes into the bowl of it, through which you must blow into the bowels."[10] What possible reasoning led to advocate introducing smoke through the anus of a drowning person is something I fail to understand. Still, this measure was not the recommendation of a fringe group but part of the therapeutic arsenal of mainstream medicine from the 17th century to the early 19th century.

Intrarectal smoke insufflation was recommended not only for drowning victims but also as a measure against intestinal colic, incarcerated hernia, volvulus (a twisting of a segment of intestine upon itself, causing severe obstruction), and severe constipation.

Special apparatuses were constructed. The 1639 edition of a book written for English ships' doctors, *The Surgion's [sic] Mate*, by John Woodall (1556–1643), who was a physician employed by East India Company, contained instructions for building a rectal tobacco-smoke "fumigator." The book referred to the many conditions likely to afflict mariners during long sea voyages. Reanimation of near-drowned sailors was especially important at a time when few people, sailors included, knew how to swim. Some devices for rectal fumigation consisted of receptacles for the burning tobacco, joined to a flexible tube, one end of which attached to a cannula that was inserted in the patient's rectum, while the opposite end bore the mouthpiece through which the therapist blew. Alternatively, the tobacco would burn in a specially constructed clyster syringe with a very long tip, connected by its proximal extremity to a long, flexible tube, at the end of which the therapist could blow.[11]

A major treatise devoted to intrarectal therapy by Regnier de Graaf included mention of this procedure only to appropriately question its effectiveness. In our own time, when antitobacco campaigns have reduced smokers to stealthy, semiclandestine practitioners of their habit, they may wistfully agree with a modern translator of de Graaf's treatise who exclaimed, "What good news for smokers! To be able to indulge by both ends!"

The exalted position of air breathing in popular, philosophical, and medical thinking explains past efforts to revive the dead by air insufflation into the lungs. An unsubstantiated tradition has it that Paracelsus and the 16th-century French surgeon Ambroise Paré tried to do just that with fire bellows. Their subjects, of course, stubbornly resisted being brought back to life. Yet the annals of medical history contain instances of individuals who survived episodes of severe asphyxia without the benefit of artificial respiration and in circumstances that, to all appearances, should have resulted in death—none more dramatic among these than the case of Anne Green, a woman who was "resurrected" in the 17th century.[12]

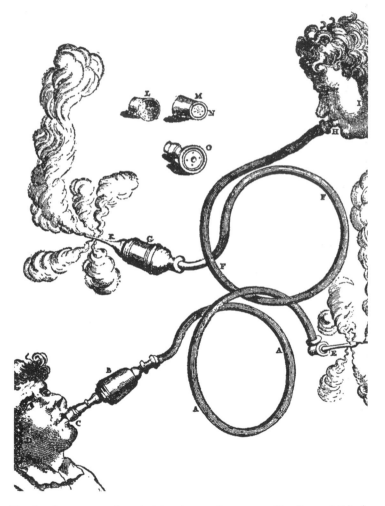

Fig. 6 Apparatuses for administering smoke enemas (*La Presse Médicale*, 1903).

Anne Green was a young woman in her twenties when she was employed as a maidservant in the house of Sir Thomas Read, lord of Duns Tew Manor, in Oxfordshire, England. Duns Tew (the word *tew* means a ridge, and *Duns* may derive from an Anglo-Saxon surname, Dunns, which first appeared in the 13th century) is now a smiling, quaint English village of stone cottages, winding roads, green lawns, and affable neighbors. However, in the 17th century it must have looked very different, marred by the prevailing lack of hygiene and stamped by the prejudices, fanaticism, and social injustice of that era. The young woman was seduced by the lord of the manor's grandson and conceived a bastard son from this union. In itself, the episode was trivial and probably not uncommon at a time when the powerful could oppress the lower classes with almost total impunity. But the events took a tragic turn: the child was stillborn, the mother tried to hide the body, the little corpse was found, and Anne Green was accused of murder, declared guilty, and condemned to death.

The penalty for a woman found guilty of killing her own son was death by hanging. In accordance with the law, the execution was carried out at Cattle Yard in Oxford on December 14, 1650. Ever respectful of tradition and legal procedure, the people of Duns Tew conducted a proper execution. The sentence was read, hymns were sung, and a distressed Anne Green, noose at her neck, was dropped from the top of the gibbet's stairs. As custom dictated, some came forward to pinch the hanged woman's breasts for amusement or to swing themselves from the suspended body, sometimes lifting it up, then hanging themselves to its legs as it fell, so as to cause a sudden jerk and precipitate the executed person's demise, thereby abbreviating what could be, at times, a painful agony.

The official executioner was upset at all these gambols. Why, with all those unruly youths swinging themselves from the victim's body, the rope might snap or be rendered useless for the next execution! Thus, he put an end to the horseplay, placed the body in a coffin, and sent it to the home of Dr. William Petty, lecturer at the university. The golden age of anatomical dissection was still at its apogee. A number of prominent physicians assembled for an anatomical demonstration, among which were doctors Ralph Bathurst (1620–1704) and Thomas Willis (1621–1675), the latter a "household name" to all physicians, on account of a group of arteries at the base of the brain that bears his name, the "Circle of Willis."

Imagine these gentlemen's surprise when, just as they were getting ready to start the dissection, they saw the "corpse" struggling to breathe and making stertorous sounds. Immediately, the combined expertise of those medical luminaries converged toward reviving the woman. They propped her up, pried her mouth open to administer hot fluids, rubbed and massaged her vigorously all over her body, applied hot bandages and compresses, and, with all the means available to medical science, tried to induce her to cough. No sooner did she begin to respond favorably than the doctors resorted to the inevitable multipurpose remedy in vogue, abundant bleeding. Thanks to their solicitous ministrations, or perhaps in spite of them, she finally came to. Twelve hours after her failed execution, Anne Green was able to say a few words; after one day, she could respond briefly to questions; two days later, she had recovered her memory, except for the events of her execution and subsequent revival; and four days later she could take some solid foods. In a month's time, she was deemed to be fully recovered.

In view of the extraordinary circumstances of the case, the local court officers solicited from higher authorities her definitive reprieve, which was granted. Having obtained her freedom, Anne Green moved with friends to Steeple Barton, about two miles from Duns Tew. She brought with her the coffin in which she had been laid to rest. She later married, had three children, and died at 31 years of age.

The torment to which she was subjected—a fall from a height of between 4 and 6 feet or 1.2 to 1.8 meters, with a rope wrapped around the neck, in the expectation that the sudden jerk would break her neck—continued to be the official manner of execution in England until the latter half of the 20th century. In time, a grim science was developed, the goal of which was to determine the appropriate height from which those executed by hanging must fall, according to the respective bodily weight. The calculation had a "humanitarian" aim: it was supposed to avoid the unnecessarily prolonged agony that occurred when the fall was insufficient to cause instant death. On the opposite extreme, too forceful a tug on the neck could cause decapitation, as when the executed was dropped from an excessive height. (This gruesome occurrence took place in Baghdad as late as January 2007, during the execution of one of the close associates of the deposed Iraqi tyrant Saddam Hussein.) In England, the last woman to be executed was Ruth Ellis, on July 13, 1955; but the last hanging, of two men, was in 1964. The British Parliament abolished capital punishment for murder in 1965, and for all crimes, both in civil and military cases, in 1998.

The Precious Air We Breathe and Its Destination

That the air we respire is life itself is an intuitive notion registered in all civilizations. Yet it was not always incorporated into a philosophical system. The Greeks, however, not only acknowledged the importance of air very early on but reflected on it with all deliberation. The earliest thinkers, the Milesians, subscribed to the notion that "all things proceed from one and are resolved into the same." Thus, the Greek philosopher Thales had proposed that all things come from water; his contemporary Anaximander, that they come from an indefinite substance which he called "the Boundless" (*apeiron*); and Anaximenes, who lived about the middle of the sixth century B.C., maintained that air was the primary substance of the universe. From air, he believed, came everything that exists, and this by a process of rarefaction and condensation: rarefied air becomes fire; condensed, it becomes wind, then cloud, then water, then earth; and when condensation is extreme, it turns into stones. Three air-derived products—fire, water, and earth—are the originators of everything else, but air is always primary; it is the mother substance in the universe.

Anaximenes realized that differences in quality are reducible to differences in quantity, a pivotal concept on which science has rested ever since. For whether we speak of light, sound, color, electromagnetism, physiology, or whatnot, all the physical phenomena, if they are to be approached scientifically, must be amenable to mathematical expression. As a scholar puts it, "only when so reduced can [they] be regarded as scientifically described."[13]

Anaximenes chose air in preference to water or earth, or some other substance, and it is easy to see why. Air is invisible, subtle, mobile, and life giving, since its brief absence suffices to hurl us down the dark abyss. The elementary imagination everywhere reckoned: if it moves by itself, it must be living. And an agent that is mobile, ethereal, alive, and life sustaining had to be divine; air was the best candidate to be the *arche*, the originator of all things.

Air being the very stuff of life and soul, it was no wonder that it was attributed fecundating powers. An ancient widespread belief was that a female could be made pregnant by the wind alone, without any need of sexual union. In the *Iliad*, the horses of Achilles were conceived when their mother, Podarge, was impregnated by the West Wind as she grazed on a meadow (XVI, 150). The Roman poet Virgil, in a celebrated passage of his *Georgics* (II, 270–276) states that mares conceive by inhaling a gentle breeze. The ancient Egyptians maintained that vultures were fecundated by the wind. As Plutarch recounted, "They say that male vultures are never found, indeed all are female, [and these] fearing scarcity of offspring . . . fly before the South wind, or if this is not blowing, spread themselves toward the East wind by opening the mouth and after three years they give birth" (*Quaestiones Romanae*, Book II, chapter 46). The story is repeated by the Roman writer Aelian, who applies it to sheep, and in addition tells us that the direction of the wind has an influence in determining the sex of the offspring. These ideas were current for a long time, and accepted everywhere with such credulity as to make us cringe today. No fewer than eight Church Fathers invoked them to support the biologic reality of the Virgin Birth.

We take a deep breath, and we sense the current of this marvelous air coming into our chest. Just where is this vivifying, spirit-uplifting affluence going? As every schoolchild will tell you, the air we inhale blows straight into our lungs. Few, however, will have a good representation of what this destination looks like. Those of us who do—by virtue of our job—can tell you: as soon as one cuts open the chest wall, removing the anterior part of the ribs and the sternum, the lungs appear as structures of a perfectly smooth, shiny, moist surface. This is because an even, taut, glossy membrane covers them—the pleura—which also lines the inner surface of the chest wall. It used to be that in young persons, the color of the lungs was a nice grayish pink, which turned deeper gray as the subject aged. This was because the inhaled soot and dust with carbon-containing particles accumulated slowly. No more. Today, as an effect of the polluted quality of the air in most cities, even the lungs of children may display a number of black deposits that impart to their surface a slate gray or blackish tint.

The lungs are paired organs of roughly conical shape, with the base below and the truncated, rounded apex (the highest point of the lungs) above. The apex comes up to a little less than an inch above the first rib or the inner end of the collarbone (clavicle) at the upper orifice of the chest cavity. This situation attracted the attention of some physicians in the 19th century; they thought that the lungs' apex was imprisoned and constricted by the bones that form the thoracic superior outlet, and that this thralldom made them especially vulnerable to tuberculosis. This disease was a worldwide scourge at the time, and the apex of the lung was its commonest site of onset.

The two organs weigh together a little less than a kilogram in an adult man of average build, and about three-quarters of a kilogram in a woman. Normally, the left-sided lung is smaller than the right, because it is excavated on its inner aspect, and this concavity is there to lodge the heart: it is the *cardiac bed*. The ancients, who knew little anatomy, did not ignore this detail; they concluded that the left lung wraps itself around the heart for the specific purpose of cooling it off. For the heart being the seat of the passions, the conveyor, and in the Galenic system largely the generator of heat, it was especially prone to overheating. Before "boiling blood" became a trite metaphor for a man's dudgeon, it was a literal reference to an alleged physiologic phenomenon; and William Harvey, in order to establish his epoch-making discovery of the circulation, had to contend first with claims that very little blood passed through the heart with each beat, because boiling had turned most of it into foam. An all-seeing Providence had determined that an organ so distinctly liable to overheat should be furnished with an abutting cooling system.

The ancients thought that the lung had a refrigerating physiological role. Plato wrote that when the heart swells with suspense and anger, this is acknowledged as due to fire; therefore, the gods devised relief for it by making the lung soft, bloodless, and porous, like a sponge. And so, each time the fire of the passions blazes forth and threatens the heart with overheating, the coolness of air and drink—for they thought that drinks passed through the lungs (see below)—would lower its temperature (*Timaeus* 70c).

The cooling function of the lungs was an enduring concept. Francis Bacon (1561–1626), that "glory of his age and nation, adorner and ornament of learning," as some panegyrist called him, believed that the swiftness of death in suffocation, as by strangling or drowning, is not so much due to the stoppage of lung motion "as to the stoppage of refrigeration, because air when too hot, though it be freely drawn in, is no less suffocating than if respirations were stopped." He offered as proof the death of those who died in rooms where coals are burning or a fire has been lighted. His age being still blissfully ignorant of carbon monoxide toxicity, Bacon can confidently heap the examples that reinforce his thesis: "The same happens likewise from the overheating of dry baths, as was practiced in the death of Fausta, wife of Constantine the Great."[14]

The sensation that one gets by taking a human lung into one's hands is difficult to describe. This organ is lighter than its volume may lead us to expect, since it has a large content of air. Which is why, if one drops it into water, the lung will float. Yet the lung of a stillborn baby, who never breathed, sinks to the bottom. The tactile sensation it gives reminds us of a sponge, elastic and springy. When compressed by our hand, it crackles. The cut surface, upon close inspection, reveals innumerable, minute, air-containing cavities. These, like so many bodily structures, were dignified with a noble Latin term: *alveoli*, singular *alveolus*, the name the ancient Romans gave to a tooth socket, and the diminutive of *alveus*, a channel.

Now, if one had to compare the gross appearance of this organ to any known object, the choice of a sieve would be appropriate. A sieve is a device comprised of numerous tiny holes, not unlike the pulmonary alveoli—hence, the ancient Greeks' notion that the lung had a sifting function. Alas, for all their sublime intellectual conquests, the Greeks had this one failing, that they put abstract reasoning above all else. They were prompt to follow any speculation, when it might have been better to observe the facts first, and to theorize later. As a scholar once put it, they "tried to explain Nature while shutting their eyes." They reasoned by analogy: if the organ looks like a sieve, it must work like a sieve. None other than Plato had affirmed in *Timaeus* that "what we drink makes its way through the lungs into the kidneys, and thence to the bladder ..." Why would the gods have made the lung like a sieve if its only function were to transmit air? Air needs no sieve, since it can escape from any place; therefore, the lung's structural design had to do with the passage through it of solids or liquids, or both.

Plutarch (A.D. 45–120) recounts a lively dinner discussion about this subject.[15] It all starts when one of the guests, waxing poetical after much libation, recites a verse of Alcaeus, a follower of Plato: "Wet now the lungs with wine; the dog-star shines." Upon which the physician Nicias of Nicopolis, one of the convivials, retorts: "Wet the lungs with wine? Who ever heard of such nonsense?" And he goes on to explain that the wine goes through the esophagus, not through the windpipe. This is ensured by the epiglottis, a formation strategically placed in our gullet that works as a door, opening or shutting as needed. It rises to permit the ingress or egress of breath, but closes down when we take food or drink, so that neither of these falls into the windpipe. When this accidentally happens, everyone knows the hard, distressing coughing and asphyxiation that follows. Nicias learned all this when he studied with Erasistratus of Cos, the savant who performed anatomical dissections in Alexandria, in Egypt.

But the rest of the convivials are not impressed. For one thing, this Erasistratus had a very bad reputation. Celsus, the famous physician of ancient Rome, called him a callous, unfeeling man who dissected living human beings. Although this imputation may have been made on shaky grounds, it passed for the truth on account of that human propensity to systematically believe the ill and disbelieve the good that is spoken of our fellows. The "butcher of Alexandria," the banqueters might have called him. Would the opinion of such a reprobate be placed against that of the divine Plato or Euripides, the great dramatist, or the eminent physician Philiston of Locris, or of no less an eminence than Hippocrates, the father of medicine? For all these illustrious men taught that what we drink goes through the lungs.

One of the defenders of the lung-as-sieve hypothesis then rises to make his case with a persuasive speech, which we may rephrase as follows:

"When a soldier has his throat slit in battle, some fluid oozes through the windpipe. Is this not direct proof that fluid travels to the lung? But there is more. The patient whose lung is affected by inflammation experiences an excessive, burning thirst. The dryness or the heat provokes the desire for liquid; the lung must have some liquid, since this is its normal function. Note that creatures that do not have a lung, or have a very small one, feel no need to drink, or experience only a minimal desire for liquids. And think, moreover, why is there a urinary bladder? The stomach receives both food and drink, which it conveys to the lower abdomen. You would think that the residue of these ingesta should pass to the outside through the same bodily orifice, since they travel together. Instead there are two passages: one for liquid wastes, the other for solid residues. Why? Because the former come from the lungs, and the latter from the stomach. The separation takes place at the beginning, right after we swallow, thanks to the epiglottis. For the role of this formation is not what Nicias explained, it is to divide what goes to the stomach from what goes to the lungs.

"Notice, also, that the liquid excretion is pure and uncontaminated. You would expect, if the liquid were mixed with the solid inside the abdomen, that there would be some sort of mixture or amalgamation. You would then expect to see the liquid with at least some solid particles. But the fact is that the two are quite separate: one went through the lungs, the other through the alimentary tract. This is why they look different, and we certainly know they smell different! Yet if the two went down the same route, it would be logical to expect some cross-contamination that would impart common sensible properties to the two excreta, solid and liquid.

"You say that the ingesta that go through the stomach are concentrated and solidified in the belly? Then they could just as well become solidified in the bladder. But this is not the case, for we never see solid residues in the urine. Why? Because the fluid goes through the windpipe, and as it courses through there, the stomach draws a little of it—just enough to smoothen and to liquefy the food. The bulk of the liquid enters the lung, where it is distributed, together with the air, to the parts of this organ that need it most, and all the rest is sent to the bladder."

A fine example of reasoning power unencumbered by facts! The ancient Greeks' intellect, riding roughshod the spirited steed of imagination, generated hypotheses so quaint, or explanations so colorful, that I, for one, wish they were true. They bring to mind the old Italian saying, *Se non e vero e ben trovato*, which we may freely render, "Perhaps untrue, but very nicely imagined."

Strange as it may seem, it took over 17 centuries for a rational, scientific explanation of human breathing to finally emerge. An early formulation was made by a singular English gentleman named John Mayow (1640–1679). With remarkable prescience, he wrote: "Some suppose that respiration chiefly serves for cooling the heart; but heating rather than such a cooling seems to suit the circulation and fermentation of the blood." And he added: "There is yet another use of respiration [...] Life, if I am not mistaken, consists in the distribution of animal spirits, and their supply is most of all required for the beating of the heart and the flow of blood to the brain." The formation of such "animal spirits" depended on something present in the air we breathe. In his words: "... an aerial something essential to life, whatever it may be, passes into the mass of the blood. And thus air driven out of the lungs, these vital particles having been drained from it, is no longer fit for breathing again."[16]

This "aerial something essential to life" was, of course, oxygen. Profiting from the experiments of his learned compatriot Robert Boyle (1627–1691), Mayow proposed the existence of certain particles in the air that were necessary for the lighting of a fire ("igneo-aerial" particles).

This concept was reminiscent of the speculations of the "atomist" philosophers who proposed the presence of minute, invisible corpuscles of various properties in the composition of the universe. Mayow's particles, however, were not the whole of air but only part of it; he conceived of them as fixed to niter, and therefore as existing in air as well as in gunpowder. In a series of ingenious and carefully described experiments which he illustrated himself with fine drawings, Mayow identified combustion with breathing.

He placed a lighted candle and a small animal enclosed together in a glass jar and observed that the animal lived only half the time that he would survive in the absence of the candle. This happened, he thought, because the lighted candle contributed to the exhaustion of igneo-aerial particles. Therefore, "animals and fire draw the same kind of particles from the air." He hypothesized that the union of nitro-aerial particles with combustible material throughout the body was responsible for body heat.[17]

Mayow's many remarkable insights would be confirmed, modified, or expanded, and given a scientific, quantitative format about 100 years later by the work of Joseph Priestley (1733–1803) and the ill-fated Antoine Lavoisier (1743–1794), who definitively established that oxygen is present in the air and that animals produce heat by a type of combustion.[18]

Breathing Compromise in Literature

The atomist philosophers of antiquity proposed the existence of life-giving minute particles in the air. It fell to the fathers of bacteriology in the 19th century, such men as Louis Pasteur and Robert Koch, to demonstrate the presence of death-giving particles. In each one of the minuscule, nearly invisible droplets ejected by an infected person during coughing or sneezing, travel hundreds of living microorganisms that, should we happen to inhale them, can convey the infection into our lungs.

Among modern fiction writers, the idea that life and death are linked to breath was the theme of an engrossing story by Luigi Pirandello (1867–1936). Its title, "Soffio," may be translated as "breath" or a "whiff of air." The narrative starts as the protagonist, who is the narrator and speaks in the first person singular, is approached by a friend coming to announce that a mutual acquaintance has suddenly died. His only comment on hearing the news is, "Such is life. A puff is all it takes to blow it away . . ." And he emphasizes the uttering of this commonplace with a lively hand gesture (Italian, after all, we suppose him to be): pretending to hold a feather between the thumb and index finger, he approaches these to his lips, then blows at them, as if to send the feather to the wind. To his unmitigated surprise, immediately thereafter the man who brought the sad news becomes intensely pale, places a hand on his chest, and staggers; he is nearing collapse and must be helped home. A sudden indisposition caused by recounting the story of a compeer's demise? Perhaps. But the next day the narrator learns that this friend, too, has died.

There was sufficient cause here for anxiety. One more friend appears who cannot fail to express a mixture of pain and perplexity upon learning the circumstances of the fatal episode. He utters the obligatory "But I just saw him yesterday morning, and he seemed the very picture of good health!" To which our man retorts, almost mechanically, that life is like that, flimsy and ethereal: here today, gone tomorrow. At the same time, his thumb and index finger contact each other at the tips, and the hand, almost automatically, moves toward his face. The motion is quasi-involuntary, like an automatism. But once the fingers have reached the level of his face, he feels compelled, in order not to seem ridiculous, to say "Life is like that!" and at the same time he blows, ever so lightly, on the two joined fingers while drawing them apart, as if he were releasing a feather into the wind.

Once again, no sooner is this gesture completed than his interlocutor feels suffocated and falls backward on a sofa, breathing with difficulty and turning alarmingly blue. In great haste, he is taken home to his relatives, but once there, before a physician can be summoned and to the utter despair of his inconsolable sister, he breathes his last.

How to depict the terror and the maddening confusion of a man who begins to suspect that his own breath is transformed into a lethal weapon? If this is true, he thinks, perhaps it is best to try it on himself, and end once and for all this curse that has befallen him. In a state of great agitation, he tells the bereaved sister how the accident happened, and, adding open-mouthed amazement to her disconsolateness, implores her to blow on his fingers, so that she can see how this simple act can bring death upon himself. A physician has just arrived, too late to be of any help to the deceased, and our death blower accosts him too with the same pressing request: "Just blow here, on my fingers, toward me! Blow! It is all that is needed to provoke death!"

Predictably, they think he has gone mad. The physician is used to dealing with the mentally deranged or the simply distraught by the shock of personal tragedy. He tries to appease him as best he can. Seeing that reasoning is futile, he tries humor, however ill suited to the occasion: "What! Blow and kill you? Good gracious, no! I am not about to blow a second death when we just had one by that method. One a day is more than enough!" And with these pert remarks, the medical man nimbly absconds.

The presumptive death blower is prey to growing distress. Can it be true that he has the ability to dispense death? Perhaps he is immersed in a spine-chilling nightmare from which he will soon awake, or under some delusion that will soon pass. In a distraught state, he runs out of the house and wanders through streets, alleys, and plazas. Here and there he encounters bystanders or strollers in whose direction he blows, with his fingers against his lips in the now habitual gesture, aiming indiscriminately toward men, women, and children. At last he withdraws to his bedroom, asking himself, Can he exterminate the entire city population? Could he depopulate the suburbs, the farms, the neighboring villages? Was his cursed power strong enough to wipe off the entire human race from the face of the earth? To these hectic thoughts, he falls asleep. The next day, he discovers that all the newspapers carry, in conspicuous front-page headlines, the announcement that an epidemic has hit the city, and people are dying like flies: death overtakes men, women, and children everywhere, and the public sanitary services seem insufficient to cope with the emergency.

He no longer doubts his baneful power. He metes out his lethal dispensation on those he judges unworthy of living or too grievously oppressed by the pains in their lives. But his torment only grows larger: it is beyond human endurance to adopt the role of exterminating angel. In a fit of despair, he denounces himself to a group of health care workers: a physician and some medical students and nurses that he encounters at a hospital's threshold. Alas, he meets with the anticipated derision. Angered and humiliated by their scorn, he taunts them by proposing to demonstrate his power on them. They accept, thinking that to go along with the preposterous bidding of a lunatic will do no harm and might earn them some good laughs. The merry group stands Indian file before the challenger, this one blows on them his customary puff, and straight away they totter and fall to the ground one by one, this one moaning, that one mute, wide-eyed and in a cold sweat, still another imploring mercy to the slayer. The physician, even as he bends to the floor, exclaims, "The epidemic! The epidemic!"—a skeptic and a rationalist to the very end.

The story has no conventional resolution, no denouement in the traditional sense. We do not learn whether the protagonist is a madman under a psychotic delusion, or a fictional personage in the style of Nathaniel Hawthorne's "Rappaccini's Daughter," endowed with the sinister, magical ability to kill from a distance. He withdraws to the countryside, and there, after much tortured cogitation on the dark omnipotence that has been visited upon him, concludes: "It was me, it was me. I was death; I had death between two fingers and in the breath, and I could make them all die."

This utterance suggests that Pirandello's death blower was the fictional or symbolic incarnation of an epidemic. But he seems to be more than that. For at the end of the narrative, Pirandello offers us a lyrical set piece that throws into relief the dual character, baneful and benign, of the phenomena of nature. The death blower has left the crowds of the city for the peace of the countryside. In this bucolic setting, he feels inundated by a sense of oneness with his surroundings. The slightest tremor of a grass blade when touched by an insect that alights on it is registered in the innermost fibers of his being. He observes a couple of white butterflies in amorous flight, and compares their flickering, undulating cruising to the unsteady wavering of paper bits blown by the wind. Then, he widow

. . . over there, sitting on a bench protected by oleanders, a young girl in a dress with a sky-blue veil, and a great straw hat decked with Damask roses; her eyelashes fluttered; she was thinking and smiling, with a smile that made her look distant, like an image of my youth; may be she was nothing but an image of life that still remained there, now alone in the world. One puff, and she's gone! Moved to the point of anguish by so much sweetness, I stood there, invisible, hands clasped and holding my breath, watching her from afar; and my gaze was the breeze itself that caressed her without her realizing that she was being touched.[19]

Is this not a striking image? In the fullness of youth's splendor, our feverish exultations set our souls in the rapt suspension of work, or passion, or creation. But joys and triumphs, like intense woe and sadness, render us unaware of the soft wind that blows around us. Attention: mark this caressing zephyr, this mild breeze; it is the gaze of death constantly watching us, entranced from afar—a premonition of the strong gale that is to follow, and which will bear us away in its bosom, like motes in the wind. Blown away! A puff is all it takes.

The Real Thing: Destruction Abrupt or Gradual

The fictional death spreader in "Soffio" has an apt prototype in objective reality. The patient who spreads lethal infections in the form of aerosol clouds while coughing or sneezing is its proper counterpart. When highly contagious, simple respiratory movements become the mechanism that ejects a potentially deadly spray.

And in terms of contagiousness, the most egregious example was the influenza epidemic, the famous "Spanish flu" pandemic of 1918–1920, the greatest global public health disaster ever known. About 40 million people died (by some estimates, between 50 million and 100 million): more than in the horrid hecatomb of the First World War and possibly more than in all previous wars combined. The dismal conditions of life in the trenches, forced on large contingents of men during that conflict, did much to enhance the diffusion of the disease. More people succumbed in one year of the influenza pandemic than in four years of the nefarious Black Plague that devastated Europe in the 14th century. One-fifth of the world's population was infected. The number of deaths decreased the average lifespan of Americans by ten years.

As in Pirandello's story, people died in the streets during the influenza epidemic. There were reports of men catching the disease on their way to work and dying on the job a few hours later. In a much recounted episode, a group of four women gathered to play bridge; at the end of their session, three had fallen ill and died shortly thereafter. A letter written in 1918 by a physician stationed at Camp Devens, Massachusetts, and later published in the *British Medical Journal* (December 22–29, 1979), gives an idea of what the influenza pandemic looked like from his vantage point. The soldiers were healthy young men who started with what seemed a common cold but turned into

> . . . the most vicious type of pneumonia that has ever been seen. Two hours after admission they have Mahogany spots on their cheekbones, and a few hours later you can begin to see the Cyanosis [blue discoloration] extending from their

ears and spreading all over the face, until it is hard to distinguish the colored men from the white. It is only a matter of a few hours until death comes, and it is simply a struggle for air until they suffocate. It is horrible [. . .] We have been averaging about a hundred deaths per day, and still keeping it up . . .

For all their fulminating puissance, epidemics of acute respiratory disease have been sporadic and their cyclic violence has been blunted to some extent by improved living conditions and medical advances. Historically, the major cause of devastation of the lungs was not abrupt. The chief respiratory ailment had none of the dramatic struggling for air seen in drowning, asphyxiation, or acute, rapid destruction of lung tissue. It was a slow, insidious disease that gnawed relentlessly at the substance of this organ; a disease that, in view of its enormous diffusion, merited the impressive name of White Plague: tuberculosis. During the period between the 18th and early 20th centuries, this was the leading cause of death in the Western world, for all age groups.

Suffering came not by way of an explosive aggression but in a sly, torpid guise: a persistent, dry cough in reiterative bouts, so stubborn and intense that after a meal it was often followed by vomiting; a no less inflexible, low-grade fever that came back every afternoon to bedew the patient's brow with sweat; a certain languor as its invariable concomitant; and the whole constellation of symptoms accompanied by an extenuation that sapped the body's energy while reducing its substance. The doctors gave it a cryptic-sounding Greek name, as they did to all that they did not understand and could not cure: *phthisis*, a wasting away; in other words, consumption.

Diderot's *Encyclopedia* defined phthisis as "what comes from any ulcer, which applied to the lungs or any other part, corrupts it, destroys it, and makes it fall into marasmus and shrivels it up." It was the kind of withering that allowed the consumptive to "bid a pathetic farewell to the world and prepare his/her voyage to the beyond." Therefore, it was easy to veil its tragic aspects with the trappings of theatricality, and it is not surprising that the Romantic movement, with its interest in melancholia, reverie, the mysterious, and the preeminence of sentiment over reason, should have emblazoned this pathology with all the elements of its art. The veritable epidemic of tuberculosis that swept the world during the Romantic period left in its wake a legion of "romantic phthisics": the poet John Keats (1795–1821), dead at 26 years of age, having foreseen and most poignantly announced his own end, by virtue of his medical training; the 18th-century hostess and exemplary lover Julie de Lespinasse (1732–1776), whose celebrated salon was the "research and development laboratory" for the French Revolution; the Brontë family, which gave to the world three immortal writers in the Victorian age, but in which three sisters, one brother, and their mother all succumbed to the same disease; the promising painter and ardent feminist Marie Bashkirtseff (1858–1884), cut down in her prime; and a number of others. The renowned historical patients are too numerous to mention, but the list extends into the modern age with victims as unlikely as public health benefactor Dr. Josephine Baker, New Zealand writer Katherine Mansfield, and tennis champion Alice Marble.

The Story of a Famous *Poitrinaire* (Chest Patient)

Among the men, perhaps the most famous patient with respiratory disease was a gentleman who answered to the following description: medium height; the face, an oval that seemed lengthened without being thin; the complexion, distinctly pale; a long and incurved nose; an unusually tall forehead; the hair, brown; a lower lip somewhat tumid and protuberant; his carriage, distinguished and aristocratic, an impression greatly enhanced by his invariably elegant and impeccably fashionable attire; his hands, said by all to be most beautiful, with long fingers whose softness and delicacy conflicted with their obvious strength; and his eyes large, deep, expressive, and of a color that in some countries is called chestnut brown, in English auburn, and in Polish *piwny*, which in Poland also designates the brown beer. Nor is this an idle reference, since the man was Polish, and a nationalist at that, although he lived most of his life in France, where he died. His name was Fryderyk (Frédéric in the French spelling, which he made his, and by which he became known) Chopin.

No biographer omits to speak of Chopin's torment from phthisis, or consumption. It is indeed an often-told tale, for it is generally assumed that the disease must have greatly influenced this artist's creativity. Yet there are reasons to doubt the accuracy of such a diagnosis. What cannot be doubted is that Chopin was a frail man; at least his health was a cause for worry to his family from the time he was a boy. In a letter to his parents in 1824, when he was 14, he asks permission to eat rye bread, which physicians had prohibited to him; and he describes drinking a number of infusions, presumably for reasons of health. Two years later, the circumstantial evidence has been said to be stronger: he suffers from an infected lymph node in the neck region, sometimes a characteristic feature of tuberculosis, the so-called scrofula. Note, however, that this by no means gives diagnostic certainty: a swollen lymph node may have many other etiologies. At any rate, he was subjected to the treatment that prevailed in his time, consisting of the application of leeches to the neck—and he seems to have recovered.

At the end of July 1826, on the advice of Dr. Malcz, one of his family physicians, Frédéric accompanied his little sister Emilia to a cure at Reinertz, a thermal station in Silesia (present-day Duszniki-Zdrój, near the border between Poland and the Czech Republic). One year later, Emilia died of tuberculosis. To many biographers, this evokes the hypothesis that Chopin may have suffered a contagion, but no evidence substantiates this possibility. At least, he did not manifest any suggestive symptoms or signs in the period shortly after his sister's demise.

In September 1828, young Frédéric's natural history professor, Mr. Jarocki, wished to take the 18-year-old along to a scientific congress in Berlin. Permission was granted, for the young man's many talents were already recognized by his family, his peers, and his mentors. At seven years of age, he had composed his *Polonaise in G minor*, plus a whole series of mazurkas, marches, and other airs that were played by the local band during festivities. At eight he gave his first performance as a piano soloist in a charity concert. But, although widely acknowledged as a child prodigy in music, Chopin was also gifted as a student of the sciences, especially natural history (although apparently not of mathematics). This is why it was felt appropriate to send him to the Berlin meeting, which would be presided over by Alexander von Humboldt, undoubtedly the most illustrious and revered naturalist of his time. The experience would help the young man to define his true vocation. Unfortunately for science, Chopin felt immensely bored in the midst of those learned sessions. He passed his time drawing hilarious caricatures of the attendees—another one of his many talents. His future was decided: he would devote his life to music, not to science.

A demon of activity he certainly was not. He seemed incapable of prolonged or strenuous physical effort. He tired easily. Still, in those youthful years, Chopin displayed considerable dynamism. He joined friends in political discussions, became a member of the Masonic brotherhood, attended the activities of that group, gave concerts, composed works, and started a romantic liaison with a young singer, Konstancza Gladkowska, in Warsaw. Moreover, he traveled to Vienna, then the center of the musical world; no artist who aspired to prominence in music could afford to ignore the Austrian capital. As luck would have it, only days after his departure in November 1830, the Polish rebellion against Russian domination exploded. He would never see his homeland again.

Things did not go well for Chopin in Vienna. Austria was rather hostile to the Polish cause. His concerts did not have the resonance he had hoped for, teaching jobs were neither profitable nor stimulating, and he felt painfully uprooted. The relationship with Konstancza, rather lukewarm to begin with, was further chilled by absence, until the lowering of temperature equaled zero. Homesickness added acute pangs to the young man's spleen. So he went on the road again: after giving some concerts in Germany, his roaming ended in Paris. His first impressions of the City of Lights cannot be considered wholly positive: "One finds here the greatest luxury and the greatest filth; at every step there are announces about venereal diseases," he wrote to a friend in Berlin in a letter dated November 18, 1831. "Noise, racket, bedlam, mud, more than you would think possible! [...] And how many compassionate young ladies (*demoiselles miséricordieuses*)! They pursue the passers-by."

Biographers note that the young Frédéric did not frequent the compassionate demoiselles to relieve his melancholy. Certain passages in his correspondence clearly state that he preferred to forgo their company. On the other hand, the myth of the highly spiritual young man, nearly disembodied and practically asexual, living only for the ethereal delights found in the lofty regions of art, is totally unwarranted. His correspondence also shows that he was very much in touch with the realities of everyday life and not insensible to the gravitational pulls of the flesh. "I already know some women singers, and here these seem even more desirous than those of the Tirol to make a duo," he writes to a friend. And in a postscript, he adds a savory personal anecdote:

> In the house where I am staying lives, one floor below mine, a young woman whose husband is absent from morning until very late at night. My neighbor is very pretty, and more than once she has invited me to come and console her of her solitude. There burns in her house a big fire next to which it would feel good to sit down, and she asks me to, believing that one of these days I will allow myself to be tempted.

But I have no desire to engage in these adventures. It could well be, on the other hand, that to do so would lead me to strike an acquaintance with the husband's cane.[20]

With his big brown eyes, his vast, Olympian brow, his long, flowing locks of auburn hair that contrasted strikingly with his pale complexion—and at all times elegantly attired and exuding a melancholic air—Chopin was soon *the* fashionable Parisian artist. He gave concerts, sometimes with Franz Liszt, whom he had befriended, as he had many other artists, among them Hughes Felicité Robert de Lamennais, Charles-Augustin Sainte-Beuve, Felix Mendelssohn, and Eugène Sue. He was much requested at the salons, which he preferred to the big concert halls. Financially, he did not do so well: the concerts were mainly to make himself known, but the chief source of income was the private lessons, which he was obligated to impart at the rate of about 60 present-day euros per class. Not much, considering that his distinguished students had to be received in a house furnished in high-class style, adorned with expensive gimcrackery and located in a distinguished neighborhood. And then, his carriage, his immaculate white gloves, his aristocratic clothing: assuredly, all that did cost money!

In the midst of his dizzying mundane excitement, he found occasion to enter into an amorous relationship, in Dresden, with the daughter of a Polish family of his acquaintance, Maria Wodzinska. He went so far as to formally request the belle's hand. Her parents opposed this union, perhaps because Chopin manifested a persistent cough, which at that time invariably raised the fearful specter of phthisis. Maria obediently submitted to parental authority, her letters became progressively indifferent and rarer, and Frédéric was sunk in an emotional crisis. To forget, he plunged into a whirlwind of worldly activities that only worsened his physical condition.

To his consolation, and perhaps also his misfortune, he meets the French writer Aurore Dudevant, better known as George Sand, in 1836; two years later he starts a liaison with her. She is worried by his chronic cough and enfeeblement, and has also some concerns about the health of her own two children, 14-year-old Maurice and 10-year-old Solange. She talks him into going, all four of them, to a more favorable clime. A physician comes to examine Chopin, declares that he is not phthisic, and recommends life in a sunny place. They choose the Spanish island of Majorca. At first, all seems to go well: the climate could not be better, and the travelers are in excellent spirits. They find themselves in the rural hamlet of Establiment, at some distance from Palma, the capital of Majorca. It is all very picturesque and, they think, conducive to artistic inspiration and renewed physical vigor. Unfortunately, the weather turns bad, and they are lodged in a dark, humid, cold house, penetrated by wind drafts in all directions. They had come in search of a sunny, idyllic place that would strengthen their health and uplift their flagging spirits; they find instead an uncomfortable, rude countryside that would soon turn into a nightmare.

George Sand writes to friends that the marked changes of temperature that occur during the day in that season have caused a little worsening of Chopin's health. "A little" is only a manner of speaking: the truth is that the poor man coughs and coughs ceaselessly and in a most heartrending way. Worse yet, the sputum that he raises in his violent coughing bouts is streaked with blood. Three local physicians are summoned, they examine Chopin, and all concur in the diagnosis of consumption. "One," wrote Chopin, "smelled my spit, the other hit me to find out where I spat from, the third palpated me while listening to me coughing. The first one said that I was going to burst [French *crever*, "to burst," also used familiarly for "to die"], the second that I was bursting, and the third that I had already burst."

The opinion that these two unfortunate lovebirds form of the Majorcan medical corps has to be extremely low. According to Sand, the first physician to be summoned to Chopin's bedside was a rich practitioner who deigned to make a house call for a fee nine to ten times higher than what a French colleague might have charged in comparable circumstances. After taking the patient's pulse, he declared that it was nothing and ordered some herbal infusion. By the time Frédéric's health has deteriorated to an alarming degree, Sand has already conceived the idea that physicians in these parts are a baneful, noxious, and inefficient lot. She is a highly educated woman, and the state of medicine is such that, with respect to the effects on a patient, the difference between following the dictates of a sound common sense and the prescription of a health professional is negligible. Thus, George Sand looks upon the advice of the three consultants with undisguised skepticism.

She refuses to believe her lover a phthisic, and brands the physicians ignorant and ill informed. However, they are no quacks: they are Pedro José Arabí, a member of the Royal Academy of Medicine of Palma; Bernardo Fiol, a respected and experienced physician; and Miguel Oleo, a younger colleague of the other two.[21] They make the same recommendations that any physician at the time would have made, including the most brilliant medical eminences of Paris (which, by the way, would have been as futile against the disease in Paris as in Majorca). But George Sand refuses to heed them, thinking the Spanish physicians unenlightened medicos from some backwater. Moreover, she is proud of disobeying their advice and believes this a merit on her part that will save the life of her lover.

George Sand concludes that the Spaniards, or at least the Majorcans, have "the prejudice of contagionism," and she despises them for being prejudiced. But what she sees as irrational prejudice is, in reality, well-tempered prudence. Whereas in the northern European countries, including England, Germany, Poland, and France, the contagious nature of tuberculosis was not widely accepted at that time, the Mediterranean countries, where families lived in conditions of great interpersonal proximity, had learned to fear the danger of close contact with phthisic patients. In France, the top medical expert on tuberculosis and inventor of the stethoscope, the great René Laënnec, continued to believe that this disease was hereditary and not acquired by contagion. He would die—of tuberculosis, of course—in this erroneous persuasion. George Sand, as a highly cultivated person, could be expected to adhere to the opinion of that medical eminence.

Sand and Chopin sojourned in Majorca in 1838. A little over a quarter century had to pass before clinical studies established incontrovertibly the infectious nature of tuberculosis, and nearly a half century before the discovery of the causative microbe was made by Robert Koch (1883). Yet unschooled empiricism had long taught southern Europeans to regard the disease as contagious. Thus, in Spain, King Ferdinand VI issued a decree on October 6, 1751, that ordered all physicians, on pain of severe punishments, to report every case of pulmonary tuberculosis. Following this, the mayor of each city had to order the patient's relatives "to burn all bedsheets, covers, linen, furniture, and any object of which the sick person had made use, and which might still remain on site." And this was not all. They had to "whitewash with caustic lime the whole bedroom of the patient, and to redo the floor, by removing all the floorboards or tiles of the alcove where the sick person's bed stood." Physicians who disobeyed the injunction were subject, on a first violation, to a fine, 30 days' incarceration, and a year's suspension of their license to practice. For a second infraction, the penalty doubled the jail time and added up to four years of exile. Other health personnel who willingly disregarded the decree could be sentenced to prolonged incarceration with forced labor.

These draconian measures were the only ones with which the local authorities could oppose the spread of the disease. Therefore, when the physicians appropriately reported the diagnosis they had made on Chopin, the owner of the property, a Mr. Gómez, came to ask the two guests to leave. To believe Sand, the man appeared in their presence at a moment when they were saddened by the recent deterioration of Chopin's health and vexed by the bad weather and the difficulties of their accommodation. The inopportune man aggressively declared, "in the Spanish style," said Sand, that he had learned that "we were harboring a person who suffered a disease that he found repugnant, no less and no more, [repugnant] to him, Don Gómez, the man most filthily ugly in the four corners of the earth"; that the presence of such a person was going to cause the contagion of his whole family; and that, in consequence, he ordered them to vacate the premises "in the shortest possible delay."

She went into hysterics; scarcely able to contain her wrath, she spared him no insult. In the most uncouth manner, unbecoming to a woman of her great talent and education, she riled against all the people who surrounded her, flinging epithets, slurs, and denigration on the whole Majorcan population. Chopin, always the perfect gentleman, kept a discreet silence. But they had to leave—and to pay for the furniture and the repairs to the bedroom.

They moved to nearby Valldemosa, certainly a romantic place (Chopin said of it that "no greater beauty could be wished"), but a most inappropriate one, in the middle of December, for a consumptive. No one wanted to go there, out of respect for the friars who had occupied the place until three years before, when they were expelled by a court decree and the Chartreuse (a convent of Chartreux, monks of the religious Order of St. Bruno, usually built on an isolated place) was transformed into a place of rest for visitors. There was, however, no rest for the maestro. The place was cold, humid, provided with only an old, out-of-tune piano, and people feared to approach them. This was in part fear of contagion, and in part instinctive distrust of a peasant community for this unconventional ménage. Chopin had to remain a recluse, not seen by anybody, to avoid trouble. George Sand became ever more infuriated by this ostracism, which made her insult the locals; these, in their turn, reciprocated the disparagement with their own brand of hostility toward the haughty woman.

From Sand's correspondence, it is easy to see how much she suffered in her Spanish sojourn. The peasants' dislike for the French tourists must not have been easy to bear; to the local prejudices, one must add the fact that remembrance of the harshness of the Napoleonic invasion, crueler in Spain than in other countries, was still fresh in the collective memory, and this must not have done much to enhance the popularity of the French visitors. In her vigorous, eloquent style, and with a verve that probably is not too keen about excluding a little exaggeration, Sand wrote to a friend:

> In Spain, whoever coughs is declared phthisic, and the phthisic is considered plague-stricken, infected with the mange, a leper. There are not enough canes, stones, and policemen to chase the phthisics away from every place, because according to them phthisis is catchy and therefore one must, whenever one can, kill the patient, as we smothered those with rabies two hundred years ago. What I am telling you is literally true! In Majorca we were like pariahs because of Chopin's cough and also because we did not go to Mass. My children were assaulted with stones thrown at them on the byroads. They said we were pagans and who knows what else . . .

When, in the middle of February 1839 it became necessary to transport Chopin to Palma, all hell broke loose. He had to be trundled in a two-wheeled cart, amidst untold discomfort and inconvenience. It had been impossible to rent a carriage, because it would have been necessary to burn it after usage!. The vicissitudes of this voyage worsened the musician's condition. Sand understood—at last!—that it was necessary to return to France if he was to survive. They embarked on *El Marroquín*, and during the cruise, Chopin had a most violent hemoptysis, the dramatic manifestation that Diderot's *Encyclopedia* had defined as "the ejection via the mouth of a vermilion and foamy blood coming from the lungs, and accompanied by cough and difficult breathing." It would not be his last.

He endured ten more years, wracked by the pain and distress of a relentlessly progressive chest disease. Was it tuberculosis? This has been the standard assumption of most of his biographers, mainly because this disease was one of the major health concerns in the 19th century. However, physician writers in more recent times have cast a glance at the historical evidence and point out some medical facts that cannot be reconciled with this diagnosis. For one thing, there is no "trail of contagion" in Chopin's case. Assuredly, individual resistance is quite variable, but it is remarkable that no case of tuberculosis was discovered among those who lived in the most intimate and prolonged contact with the pianist: George Sand in the first place, and then her two children, who were exposed at a particularly susceptible period of their lives. Among Chopin's closest friends and the physicians who looked after him, no one seems to have contracted the disease. Moreover, except during rare episodes of what may have been intercurrent infections, there was no evidence of fever. This remarkable feature so intrigued Chopin's physicians, that the artist mentioned it in his letters. The absence of fever in his case, he once remarked, "disconcerted and bothered the ordinary physician." His clinical evolution was not that of a progressively debilitating, chronic, and febrile infective disease, as tuberculosis typically is.

The presence of blood in the sputum is a feared, ominous sign of tuberculosis. Its dramatic impact needs no reemphasis. At a distance of about 60 years, the writer of these lines has forgotten everything about a film based on Chopin's life that he watched as a child (one of the early Technicolor films), but he still remembers a scene in which the camera focused on the ivory keys of the piano as they were suddenly reddened by the crimson blood ejected from Chopin's lungs during a violent coughing spell—this scene rendered all the more gripping by the solemn, intense music that he played and had to interrupt abruptly. But this dramatic manifestation is not exclusive to tuberculosis. Any disease that causes destruction of lung tissue (viral, fungal, or bacterial infections, sarcoidosis, tumors, bronchiectasis, and so forth) may be accompanied by bleeding. In particular, the cause of pulmonary bleeding may reside outside of the lungs, in the heart. Deficient cardiac function, by causing blood to damn up small lung vessels and excessive engorgement of the same, may lead to rupture of their delicate walls and bleeding manifested as hemoptysis.

It cannot be gainsaid that many of the features of Chopin's life accord well with the hypothesis that he was a cardiac patient. Especially noteworthy is his easy fatigability, which seems to have been present since childhood. A myth that has thrived around his personality is that of the romantic artist of ethereal aspirations and refined proclivities, delicate of mind and feeble of body. But Chopin was not one to lapse easily into mawkishness. Nor was he the dreamer, the stargazer obsessed by his art, or the idealist whose head-in-the-clouds attitude removed him from earthy concerns. Quite the contrary: a canvassing of his life, his writings, and his utterances leaves the impression that his aloofness was far from voluntary. He would have liked to engage in the many worldly activities that solicited his attention. He did as much as he could while he could: traveled, gave concerts, cultivated amorous liaisons, engaged in politics, and so on. His soul was brimming with the desire to compose and to play his music when he no longer had the strength to hold the plume or strike the piano keys. He was obligated to cut short these many activities, not willingly, but because his strength failed him, his physical stamina abandoned him, and his breath was woefully insufficient. Earlier on, his shortness of breath was episodic and asthmalike; later he had to be carried up one flight of stairs (alas, most Parisian apartments were, and many still are, located on the upper level of buildings without an elevator) in the arms of Daniel, his faithful servant of many years.

Assuming that Chopin was a cardiac patient, one wonders about the nature of the hypothetical cardiopathy. It is unlikely to have been valvular disease. He was examined by the most competent physicians at a time when Parisian doctors were cultivating the use of the stethoscope with unexampled meticulousness. They were quite capable of diagnosing valvular disease, and the same may be said for most major congenital heart diseases. However, then as now, the cardiac muscle may be the seat of various forms of pathology of unknown cause (cardiomyopathies) that may first manifest in the young and progress to end fatally in later years. Such a possibility may not be easily ruled out. It has also been suggested that a constrictive pericarditis (inflammation of the membranous tissue that surrounds the heart) could have occurred, for this disease may cause compression of the heart while accompanied by such muted chest signs as might have escaped detection with the diagnostic means available during Chopin's life.[22] But since tuberculosis is one known cause of pericarditis, this raises the possibility that the great artist may have suffered from disease in both the heart and the lungs. We must conclude that "retrospective diagnosis" is generally an unrewarding task, and that, with respect to Chopin's diagnosis, the prudent course is to abstain from too dogmatic an opinion.

In George Sand's country house at Nohant, Chopin enjoyed some placid summers that redounded to his enhanced artistic productivity. This was one of the most productive periods of his life. His immense talent earned him fame and the protection of the powerful, but, as often happens, not financial ease: he was forced to continue giving private lessons, concerts, and recitals that required great expenditure of his waning energy. It was with superhuman effort that he managed to appear in public. But there were no effective "cures" for consumption, assuming this was the correct diagnosis, and his health inexorably declined, despite the attentions of some of the most renowned physicians of the time, such as Dr. Jean Cruveilhier (1791–1874).

Finally, on October 12, 1849, in his new apartment on Place Vendôme, surrounded by a few friends, his sister Ludwika (who had overcome many obstacles to travel from Poland in those tempestuous times, to console her poor brother), his protectress Princess Czartoryska, and Dr. Cruveilhier. A rift had occurred between him and George Sand the year before; she no longer shared his life, and she was not present. Chopin received the last sacraments of the church, and, conscious to the last, his life was extinguished at two o'clock in the morning on the 15th day of that month.

Among his papers a note was found enjoining his survivors to make sure that his body was opened, for fear of being buried alive, a widespread terror in the Romantic era. Cruveilhier himself must have done this; and although a regular autopsy was not requested— and would have been considered a sort of profanation—it is difficult to believe that this physician refrained from examining the thoracic organs. This was the era of the ascendancy of anatomical pathology. It was understood at the time that this medical specialty, as its name implies, recognized and explicated the diseases through the structural modifications imprinted on the organs affected. It had just received a mighty impulse in Germany, with the work of Rudolf Virchow (1821–1902) and his collaborators, who applied microscopy and the newly developed chemical dyes to the study of pathologic lesions. Cruveilhier was among the major introducers of this discipline into France, the founder of the society of anatomical pathology in his country, and the first titular head of this discipline at the University of Paris in 1836. These antecedents make it hard to believe that some form of diagnostic examination of Chopin's organs was not done.

Historians say that an anatomopathologic report was prepared by Cruveilhier, which presumably established the presence of tuberculosis that extended to the heart and its pericardial covering. It is also said that this report was destroyed during the civil disturbances of the Paris Commune in 1871. Another version states that Cruveilhier told Chopin's sister that he "was more sick of the heart than of the lungs," but, unfortunately, there is no written document to support this version.

There was a solemn funeral ceremony at the Madeleine church; the body was buried in the Père Lachaise Cemetery. George Sand attended neither. Then, a detail of unquestionable romantic flavor was added: the heart of the artist, removed during the opening of his body, was transported to Poland, Chopin's birthplace. He never returned to his native land during his lifetime, but his affection for it was undimmed, and the return of his heart posthumously signified the steadfastness of this love. It was deposited (tuberculous pericarditis and all, perhaps?) in a silver urn that was placed in a niche excavated in a pillar of the Holy Cross Church on Krakowskie Przedmieście Street in Warsaw. The church was bombed and destroyed in the Second World War, but the relic remained intact. The temple was rebuilt and the heart restored to its former resting place.

Of Rales, Crackles, and Wheezes

No physician in the world could cure tuberculosis in Chopin's time. Rest in the countryside, clean air, and lots of sun seem to have been universal recommendations. Vacations by the sea or the mountains, or prolonged sojourns in a benign climate, may have furnished some relief, but the disease was not arrested. Those for whom such amenities were out of reach resorted to whatever measures their innocent faith, folk medicine, or ignorance and despair counseled them. In a touching short story by the Chinese writer Lu Hsün (1861–1936), a tuberculous child is given to eat bread soaked in the blood of a recently executed man.[23] Apparently this folk remedy was still common in China at the start of the 20th century. It did not work, and the poignant narrative concludes with a scene in which the mother visits the tomb of her dead child, which happens to be next to that of the executed blood donor.

But if physicians of that age could not cure tuberculosis, they observed it with unparalleled attentiveness. One of them, in particular, canvassed every aspect of this plague with admirable precision and peerless discerning power. His name was René-Théophile-Hyacinthe Laënnec (1781–1826), a Frenchman and a Breton, who pursued his pathfinding medical studies with all the tenacity of his race. Of him it has been said that he pioneered "that great

transformation whereby medicine passed, in less than two centuries, from the state of a mostly tentative art to that of a frequently exact science." His passion was to systematically confront the
signs and symptoms evinced by living patients against the lesions
found on examination of cadavers. He was, therefore, one of the
founders of the clinicopathologic method, a modus operandi that
has proved to be one of best ways for obtaining new knowledge
in clinical medicine. We see him in an oil painting by Théobald
Chartran (1849–1907). Here Laënnec is applying his ear directly
against the naked chest of a male patient during his rounds at the
Necker Hospital of Paris.

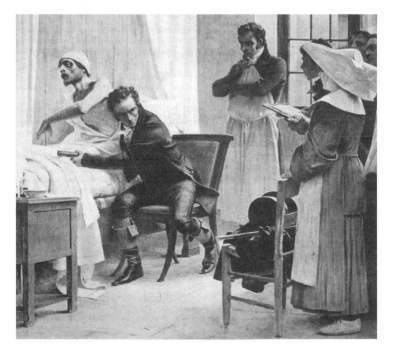

Fig. 7　Dr. René-Théophile-Hyacinthe Laënnec auscultating a patient in a
painting by Théobald Chartran. Courtesy of the National Library of
Medicine.

A physician in a white apron stands next to him, in the pensive and respectfully watchful attitude of a disciple. On the right side of the painting is a nun-nurse, coiffed in the white, starched, wide-winged headdress characteristic of her religious order. And behind her, we can descry the heads of several medical students who observe the proceedings at a distance. But the focal point remains the patient's examination. Chartran captured the physician's uncommon look, a striking alloy of nervous intensity and physical frailty. Laënnec, too, was a consumptive who would die in his forties. Here he somehow conveys an impression of intelligence, curiosity, and unswerving determination. In his left hand is a tube-like object. It is the early version of his invention, the stethoscope. A simple wooden tube! It seems ridiculously trivial by the light of today's wonders of biotechnology. Yet this trifle, this absurdly primitive device, was the keystone on which modern cardiology and pneumology were built.

What is he listening to? The whole symphony of intrathoracic disease, a music difficult to understand. Fewer and fewer physicians today cultivate this expertise. They have at their disposal a prodigiously powerful technology that informs them of the status of the inner organs, and they tend to rely on it more and more. In consequence, auscultation, although still a major component of a patient's physical examination, gradually becomes a lost art. Ironically, it has never been easier to learn it: present-day technology furnishes excellent recordings of every conceivable sound generated inside the chest.

In Laënnec's time, the clinician had to train his auditory skills to the utmost. In his *Treatise on Mediate Auscultation*, first published in 1819, Laënnec describes with exquisite prolixity every sound and sonorous nuance that is detectable with his "cylinder." Let us glance at a tiny part of his inventory. For him, a rale is not merely a rale, it is a complex sound of which there exist four distinct varieties: the humid, or crepitant; the mucous, or gurgling; the dry-sonorous, or snoring; and the sibilant, or whistling.[24] The crepitant rale, heard in pleuropneumonias, is "comparable to the noise one hears when compressing a healthy lung with one's hands." (Laënnec assumes that every clinician is or has been an autopsy dissector who knows what crushing a lung manually feels like, and how it sounds.) The mucous, or gurgling, rale is produced by the passage of air through accumulated secretions in the trachea or major bronchi: "It is the rale of dying persons, and I cannot give a more precise description. It is the only rale that can be heard with the unaided ear [in other words, without the cylinder], and then only when it originates in the trachea and main bronchi."

The dry-sonorous, or snoring, rale "resembles now the snoring of a sleeping person, now the sound that gives off a bass-viol's string rubbed with the finger, and quite often the cooing of a turtle dove. This may be so close an imitation, that one is tempted to believe that a turtle dove hides under the patient's bed."

Lastly, "the dry sibilant, or whistling, râle has varied characteristics: it may resemble a prolonged whistle, low- or high-pitched, dull or sonorous; in contrast, other times the sound is of very short duration, and resembles the tweet of little birds, or the sound emitted by two marble plaques that were smeared with oil and are brusquely separated from each other; or the noise of a little safety-valve. These different varieties of the sibilant râle exist often in different parts of the lung, or succeed each other on the same place at more or less long intervals."[25]

In an extraordinary novel entitled *Palinurus of Mexico*, a veritable tour de force of unbridled imagination, orgiastic imagery and baroque, torrential prose by the contemporary Mexican writer Fernando del Paso,[26] the author (who in his youth was a medical student) imagines a hospital ward in which the patients are classified by the sound they produce. A guide conducts an imaginary visiting physician through this area and proudly points out that they have concentrated there, "besides the classic trio formed by the patients with asthma, bronchitis and emphysema," a number of other sonorous pathologies, not the least of which are children with whooping cough and diphtheric laryngitis. There are patients with croup, whose breathing sounds are comparable to those of a flag flapping in the wind, and others whose stertorous sounds, recovered by the stethoscope, are "like those produced by a tuft of hair rubbed with the fingers"—an apt simile consigned, in fact, to textbooks of clinical medicine. Then there are those whose pulmonary sounds remind the listener of the time "when he used to blow into a soapy pipe, and then went to the park to skate and to eat cotton candy." The visitor is shown, among many other curiosities, patients who maintain a dialogue speaking with alternating grave and high-pitched utterances—a strange manifestation due to compression of the recurrent nerve, which controls the movements of the vocal cords, in turn caused by an aneurysm of the aorta. The visitor also sees patients whose thoracic sounds are reminiscent of the notes emitted by the piccolo, the flute, or the fife. For it is to be noted that certain cardiac murmurs have been termed "musical" in medical textbooks.

In del Paso's wildly imaginative novel, before the visitor leaves the hospital's "Acoustic Pavilion," he is admonished by his guide to keep in mind that all the sounds that are produced inside the body—all those whizzes and crackles, those sounds that seem caused by bellows, the tympanic sonorities that come from the abdomen; in sum, all those bodily sonorities—are there to remind us, among other things, that we are beings made of flesh and blood as well as air and gasses, and that no matter how high we pretend to soar in our intellectual endeavors, we are doomed to carry with us our constant "load of the dins and clicks and rumblings of our viscera and our cartilages." Nothing, indeed, can avoid that, even as we engage in the most ethereal or spiritual act, we should hear now and then that splashing sound produced by liquid in our digestive organs, which people vulgarly may term "noise of the tripes."

There is every appearance that, some day soon, the traditional auscultation of the chest in medical practice will become a thing of the past. In its place, there probably will be some sort of technological recording of unerring precision and high informative value. But Laënnec's perceptiveness will remain a landmark in the history of medicine. From the distance ratios between the planets, the Pythagoreans inferred a harmonious music produced by their gyrations in the cosmos, the "music of the spheres." Laënnec taught us that there is a well-accorded sonance, of which we are usually unaware, in that microcosm which is the human body; and that it breaks down into all manner of dissonance, or of new, unheard-of melodies as death approaches.

Chuang-tzu, the Taoist Chinese philosopher, left us a profoundly moving text, full of symbolic meanings, in which he contrasts the human breath blowing on reed flutes to the breath of the Great Mass of the earth. The wind, he says, is the breath exhaled by this Great Mass. When it rises, all the cavities start howling. Have you heard these bellows? he asks. In the gorges and the gullies of a mountain forest, there grow gigantic trees whose hollows are like nostrils, like mouths, or like ears; now square, now round like a bowl or a mortar; here like a wet footprint, there like a large puddle. As the wind blows through them, they growl, cry, moan, wail, shout, bellow, and emit sounds that are like those of fretted water or an arrow whiz; a little harmony when the gentle breeze blows, and a great one when a furious gale surges.[27]

Thus, Chuang-tzu presents to us the old idea of the human body as compendium or epitome of the macrocosm. And just as the gentle breeze of the normal breath provokes a small, regular harmony, the violent turbulence of disease and pulmonary disarray brings forth a multifarious dissonance, a baffling, inharmonious cacophony of gurgles and wheezes, which Laënnec strove to understand and to interpret. But there is one more sound, which the likes of Laënnec learned to identify and to fear. It is the "death rattle," the agonic stertor caused by air flowing in and out through phlegm and secretions that the dying person is too weak to cough, spit out, or swallow. This is the last sound, and those surrounding a terminal patient know it is the last. Following this, no more sonorities are heard; not even with a stethoscope.

When the fierce gusts have passed, remarked Chuang-tzu, all the cavities, crevasses, and grottos will remain empty and as silent as before. Just so, when the life-giving breath shall stop its regularly alternating inflow-outflow currents, our body will lose all its motions, like a tree whose branches and foliage stop bending and balancing when the wind subsides, and its apertures and hollows shall fall into the undisturbed, sempiternal silence of death.

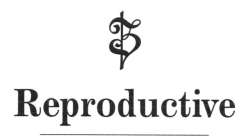

Reproductive

Part I: Female

Our First Domicile and Its Architecture

As soon as the fantastic notions of past ignorant ages were discarded in favor of the first correct concepts of human anatomy, the attention of the learned turned toward the uterus. This is the place where the portentous process of embryo formation takes place. Not in vain did the Jewish philosopher Philo (13 B.C.–CA. A.D. 50) refer to it with the high-sounding appellation *ergasterion physeos,* "the shop of nature." Inside this "shop," new human beings are fashioned; this fact alone made it worthy of the closest scrutiny.

For *Homo sapiens's* major sin has always been pride: the humblest member of our species is intimately persuaded that the Almighty had him or her in mind while achieving creation. If the universe has a purpose, maintains a claim as flattering as it is widespread, it can only be to satisfy the needs of human beings. This being so, it was logical to expect that the place where we are made, the shop of nature, should be nothing less than sublime and sumptuous.

Huge disappointment! Instead of elegant, palatial surroundings, our first cradle is the uterus, a rather prosaic, hollow viscus of thick muscular walls; an organ roughly shaped like an inverted cone, flattened from front to back and narrowed a little below its midportion by a circular isthmus that separates the cervix below from the body of the uterus, or fundus, above. Some anatomists compared its shape to that of an inverted gourd or pear: wide at the top and narrow at the bottom. Soranus of Ephesus, the foremost obstetrician and gynecologist of antiquity (born in the second half of the first century A.D.), wrote that it resembled a "cupping vessel,"[1] but this amounts to the same thing, for a Roman medicinal cup was gourdlike or pyriform. Indeed, to Hippocrates it looked like a "vessel" or a "jug" (*Epidemics*, II, 6, 5), and whoever authored the treatise on *Generation* in the *Corpus Hippocraticum* compared the womb to a vase capable of shaping the embryo, but also of deforming it, if the uterus happened to be misshapen or too small and constraining.[2]

It is said that the Roman emperor Nero, having caused the death of his mother, Agrippina, wished to see her cadaver opened because he was curious "to see the place he had come from." One of the incunabula kept at the Bibliothèque Nationale of Paris, dated from 1450, contains an illustration of the ghastly scene as imagined by a medieval artist. Agrippina's corpse lies on the dissection table, intestinal loops protruding from the incision that a dissector, a knife still in his right hand, has just performed. The emperor and another personage have come to inspect the cadaver and approach the table, while the dissector recedes, out of respect for the emperor's person—and, one might guess, out of prudence, since to keep one's distance from the likes of Nero was eminently advisable. All the figures appear anachronistically attired in medieval clothes. A tradition says that Nero "admired his mother's naked body," thereby adding a troubling note of incestuous fantasizing to the many morbid delusions of the emperor's pathologic mind. But no chronicler says whether he contemplated his dead mother's uterus or what his reaction was to the spectacle of the exposed maternal entrails.

Had he looked at "the place he came from," we may rightly suppose his frustration. There is precious little to see in the human uterus with the unaided eye. If one cuts it lengthwise or across, the central cavity will be shown to be extremely reduced. When there is no pregnancy, it looks like a mere fissure. However, on a frontal section, the cavity appears triangular, of upper base and lower vertex, the two upper angles corresponding to the entrance of the Fallopian tubes. Its capacity is no more than three or four milliliters in the virginal, adult state, or five to six if previous pregnancies have occurred. In the nonpregnant state, the cavity is virtual, since the anterior and posterior uterine walls almost touch each other; all that may be found inside it is a little mucus.

Add to this modest appearance a most unfortunate topography: a bag of urine in front, a repository of excrement behind.

The uterus is placed between the bladder and the rectum. As a piece of real estate, the uterus would be much devalued by the condition of the neighborhood. This is certainly no place of origin to satisfy the pride of men who fancied themselves sons of gods and who proclaimed their own divine nature in official ceremonies of deification, as some kings and emperors of the ancient world were wont to do. Yet the uterus is our first lodging. High and low, the meek and the exalted, our origins are always lowly: embryonic life, like death, is a Great Equalizer.

The humble appearance of this organ is so unprepossessing that the ancients underestimated its protective powers. A finer fortress could not have been built to shelter our earliest beginnings, but men of past ages adjudicated it feeble and imperfect. The uterus is a marvel of biology with amazing powers that modern science has just begun to understand. At no point in our lives are we better protected than when we inhabit this extraordinary maternal organ. Not only does it offer mechanical protection, but the subtler forms of cellular function are here displayed wholly for the benefit of the fetus. The uterus has been called an "immunologically privileged" site, because the mother's immune system, so swift to reject any foreign material, somehow tolerates the presence of the fetus (who, make no mistake, is at least half-foreign, since half of its genes come from the father). But our ancestors knew nothing of these amazing uterine strengths. They thought that a simple sneeze during copulation could dislodge the embryo from its niche inside the womb; they were convinced that mere inconvenient odors, like the smell of lamps being put out, could trigger an abortion. This inspired Pliny the Elder (A.D. 23–79) with the following rhetorical tirade:

You who put confidence in your bodily strength, you who accept Fortune's bounty and deem yourself not even her nurseling, but her offspring, you whose thoughts are of empire, you who when swelling with some success believe yourself a god, could you have been made away with so cheaply? (*Natural History*, Book VII, vii, 42)

Unimpressive and misjudged as this organ was, here is where Agrippina bore her monstrous son, although, truth to tell, she was no angel herself. To believe the Roman historian Tacitus, she precipitated her own fall by arrogantly oppressing the senate and exerting an unwholesome domination over her emperor son. Her unchecked ambition earned her a number of vindictive foes. In order to retain her power, Agrippina would balk at nothing. She was seen all made up and doing evilly sensual caresses to her inebriated son, "ready for incest," says Tacitus, except that her intentions were thwarted by intriguers who persuaded Nero to oppose her. They did not imagine that the emperor's hatred would grow to the level of wishing to murder his own mother.

He first tried to poison her. But poisoning was then a highly prevalent manner of disposing of one's enemies, and Agrippina, believing herself at risk, had the foresight to keep a good supply of antidotes handy. As it was said of the Central Asian king Mithridates, that he became immune to poison by taking progressively higher doses of venom as days went by, so Agrippina "mithridatized" herself well and good: had a venomous snake bitten her, our sympathies would have been best directed to the reptile as the likelier one to perish.

The next plan was worthy of a present-day secret agent. It was conceived by Anicetus, a former slave with engineering skills and a penchant for intrigue, who had his own reasons to hate Agrippina. He said a boat could be constructed in such a way that, once in the open sea, it would come apart and sink. Agrippina was to see the end of her days in a shipwreck, and there would be no one to blame.

The ingenious plan was put into action: a boat was made with a loose midsection, so as to give way when the sailors in the conspiracy, who themselves had the means to reach safety, would cause heavy weights to fall upon it. Nero invited his mother to a dinner in his mansion at Baiae, on the coastline, ostensibly to smooth out all differences between them; after all manner of touching protestations and filial embraces, he provided the sumptuously decorated boat that would take her back home—the rigged boat, of course. When the emperor's mother left, he saw her off, embracing her lovingly and looking tenderly into her eyes, either as a last piece of heinous deceit or because, as Tacitus generously puts it, "even Nero's brutal heart was affected by the last sight of his mother, going to her death."

Who would believe that this tortuous strategy would prove as ineffectual as the others? The lead weights were released at the proper time, crushing to death some of Agrippina's attendants, while she was preserved by the sides of the couch on which she was lying. In the confusion of the shipwreck, the killers confused Aceronia, Agrippina's friend, with Agrippina herself, and slew her. Nero's mother, to whose many wiles one must add natatory prowess, was able to swim to safety.

The treacherousness of the invitation, the contrived nature of the ship's collapse, and the deceitfulness of her son's actions became obvious to her. Nero, upon hearing of the plan's failure, was terrified. He quickly made up his mind that the best and only way to exterminate his resourceful mother was the old-fashioned way: by direct, no nonsense, bloody assassination. Accordingly, he sent murderers armed with daggers, swords, and clubs to take her life. The first to strike her was a naval captain who hit her in the head with a truncheon. She still had the strength to cry out, as another of the assassins was drawing his sword, "Strike here!" while pointing at her womb. Blows then rained upon her and she died.[3]

"Strike here!" were her last words. Presumably, she meant to say that the womb that harbored a hateful matricide deserved prompt and pitiless destruction. To believe Tacitus, astrologers had predicted her end, telling her that Nero would become emperor and then kill her. To which she allegedly replied, "Let him kill me, provided he becomes emperor!" A worse example of disproportionate ambition scarcely could be found.

Nero never heard Soranus speak, since the emperor lived from the years A.D. 37 to 68, and the physician flourished in the second century, but he must have been aware of the teachings of Soranus's professor Herophilus of Alexandria, a major figure in the history of medicine and one of the few anatomists who performed dissections in antiquity. One wonders what may have been Nero's preconceived ideas about the uterus. Curiously, the clay figures shaped as uteruses that Roman women used as ex votos in hope of curing from some uterine malady, represent this organ as girded by a series of transverse circular bands or rings, presumably made of muscle, but such annular structures do not exist. Soranus added the quaint detail that in women who have had no children, the uterus has a soft and spongy consistency, comparable to that of the tongue; but in women who have borne children, it has become more callous in consequence of repeated parturitions, and then it feels "like the head of an octopus."[4]

Soranus also quoted a less well-known author, the physician Diocles of Carystos, as having said that the interior of the uterus contains protuberances similar to breasts. These formations, broad at the base and progressively narrow at the tip, were "providentially created by nature, in order that embryos acquire the habit of sucking the nipples of the breast." This must have been a widespread belief in Greco-Roman antiquity, since it is quoted by authoritative authors such as Hippocrates (*Aphorisms* V, 45), but Aristotle, like Soranus, forcefully denied it. Wrote the Stagirite: "Those who say that children are nourished in the uterus by sucking some lump of flesh or other are mistaken," since, among other things, the embryo is surrounded by membranes that would impede such manner of nourishment.[5]

No less fanciful was the idea that the cavity of the uterus was divided into seven cells or compartments. Precisely seven, no less and no more: three on the right side, three on the left, and one in the middle. The medieval persuasion was that embryos forming on the right side were males, those on the left were female, and those who happened to take their origin in the middle chamber were hermaphrodites. Did the prospective parents desire to have a boy? Then it seemed advisable to lie on the right side during and after the sexual act. Likewise, left-sided recumbency was preferred by those—surely less numerous—who wished to beget a daughter.

This belief persisted to the Renaissance and beyond: fathers-to-be would tie the right or the left testicle while engaged in sex, in accordance with the gender they wished to impart to their offspring. The theoretical basis of this belief was rooted in Hippocratic "humoral" medicine: males developed on the right side because this is the side of the liver, which is warm and humid—the attributes of maleness. In contrast, the left side is the side of the spleen, which is cold and dry, characteristic female qualities that the spleen promptly communicates to its surroundings by organic "sympathy." Under this influence, the left side of the uterus was bound to promote the birth of females.

Just How Many Tenants per House?

The idea that parents could determine the gender of their offspring could have been served just as well by proposing only three inner uterine chambers: right, left, and middle—for embryos male, female, and neutral or composite, respectively. That the existence of seven chambers was hypothesized is a curious fact that could not have failed to attract the attention of scholars. The explanation commonly advanced is that the number seven occupied a very large place in the mind of the ancients.[6] Septenary concepts are prominent in a number of works bequeathed to us by antiquity. Solon, the celebrated Athenian poet and statesman of the sixth century B.C., is reputed to have written a poem on the "seven ages of man." Incidentally, he was one of the "seven wise men" venerated by antiquity, and although the listed sages vary, Solon's name is always among the seven. It was commonly believed that during the formation of the embryo, it took seven days for the semen to become flesh; that the menstrual flow lasted seven days; that the seventh day was critical in the resolution of any acute disease; and that seven-month fetuses were viable, whereas those eight months old were not. It was pointed out that there are seven orifices in the head and seven kinds of excretion.

Even Holy Scripture was invoked to reinforce the importance of the number seven: the Old Testament speaks of seven sons of Japheth, and ancient sources claimed that Adam had seven sons. But the arguments that passed for being most "rational" among ancient commentators were of two kinds. The first referred to the maximal capacity of the uterus. How many embryos could it hold? In general, people believed that triplets could be considered normal, but beyond that number, multiple gestations were portentous. The indefatigable and irrepressible Pliny the Elder, however, says that Egyptian women had to be excepted, because drinking the waters of the Nile made them unusually prolific. Thus, whereas in Ostia a woman named Fausta was delivered of quadruplets and this "unquestionably portended the food shortage that followed," in Egypt the same occurrence would have had no ill effects. In fact, adds Pliny, he has it from a writer named Trogus that an Egyptian woman gave birth to septuplets (". . . *in Aegypto septenos uno utero simul gigni auctor est Trogus*").[7]

Could women actually bear more than three fetuses at the same time, and this without intervention of some supernatural agency? The question was more than academic: the legal consequences could be far from negligible. Imagine a controversial lawsuit during the Middle Ages: a rich man dies, leaving a bountiful inheritance to his heirs. Seven claimants of the same age appear, asserting that they are all brothers and sisters. A decision must be made about the proper distribution of the inheritance, but here the jurisconsults will have to defer to the opinion of medical authorities. Unfortunately, the opinion of the physicians is divided.

Suppose that Mondino di Liuzzi (1275–1326), medical professor at Bologna, who left his name in the history of medicine as one of the pioneers in anatomical dissection, is called as an expert witness in the case. He firmly believes in the possibility of septuplets because he has read of its occurrence in the revered works of ancient masters and would not fail to quote Pliny in his support. Now assume that the expert witness is Pietro d'Albano (1257–1315), a physician contemporary of Liuzzi. In that case, the outcome would be quite different; for d'Albano, like his colleagues at the celebrated medical school of Salerno, not only doesn't believe in the possibility of septuplets but ridicules the very thought of such an occurrence and considers the reports of such cases as so many tall tales unworthy of the attention of serious scientists. This expert no doubt would invoke the name of Galen, whose sayings were dogma in Western medicine for over a thousand years, and who described the existence of two "concavities" in the uterus. From this, d'Albano would conclude that twins are normal, triplets exceptional, and a higher number of simultaneous gestations simply impossible, unless as miraculous, preternatural occurrences.

Today the matter is settled. Upon the advent of in vitro fertilization, which for a time thrived in a total absence of regulatory legislation, it was customary to implant a large number of embryos (despite the fact that multiple gestations had long been known to seriously endanger the lives of mother and fetuses) in the wombs of women who turned to this medical technique for the treatment of infertility. It was then shown that septuplets could come to the world, however cramped, with only the intercession of human ingenuity—no need to invoke supernatural forces. Thus, in the 1990s, the mass media disseminated the news of septuplets born here and there. On December 20, 1998, Nkem Chukwu, a Nigerian immigrant in America, surpassed all the preceding records by giving birth to octuplets. The press saluted all these events with the buoyant enthusiasm reserved for the arrival of new life and the conquests of medical science. That one of the babies died and the seven surviving siblings had to stay in the hospital for six months was evidently deemed less newsworthy; and that the quality of life of markedly premature infants is not uncommonly marred by direful complications is a fact that the world press treats with considerably less fanfare and exultation.

The ancients' second line of supposedly "scientific" argumentation was grounded in direct observations. They theorized that the number of mammillae in female animals is an indication of the number of offspring that their womb could support. In the case of human beings, however, the sow served as the model because the pig's internal anatomy was considered to exhibit the greatest similarity to the human's. (Galen's well-known use of pigs for his anatomical dissections must have weighed heavily on the minds of medieval physicians.) The sow has seven nipples (an uneven number? Or is it on each side? But this was somehow overlooked). Seven, therefore, seemed again the maximum possible number of simultaneous human gestations.

But the most curious pseudoscientific reasoning in support of the septenary concept applied to human reproduction was owed to Nikomachos, a philosopher who lived in Arabia in the second century of our era. Semen, he said, is ejaculated in seven spurts during a single coitus.[8] It was thus perfectly "logical" that there should be seven divisions in the uterine cavity and that the maximal number of births allowed by nature at one time should also be seven.

Our First Domicile a Living Animal?

It is generally known that men of past ages believed the uterus could move around in the abdomen. The origin of this stunning idea is unknown, but it had been present in the popular imagination for some time before renowned philosophers spoke about it. Yet it is often attributed to Plato, who famously granted to the uterus a sort of independent will, able to displace itself every which way inside the body and to "obstruct the passages of air, impede respiration, thus subjecting the body to the worst sufferings, and causing in it all sorts of illnesses" (*Timaeus:* 91c). In all fairness, Plato had also considered the phallus a sort of willful creature "deaf to the voice of reason, and carried away by its furious appetites."

Aretaeus of Cappadocia (fl.140 A.D.) most vividly depicted the womb's faculty of locomotion when he wrote that

> . . . the uterus, this feminine organ, is almost like an animal, for it moves by itself here and there toward the flanks; it directs itself now to the upper parts under the cartilage of the sternum, now toward the ribs, to the right or to the left,

toward the liver and the abdominal viscera, or more willingly toward the inferior parts; to say it in one word, it is an
entirely vagabond organ. It is pleasantly affected by the good
odors, and goes after them; the bad ones it suffers badly, and
flees from them. In sum, the womb in the woman is like one
animal inside another one.[9]

Thus, the sages of old followed Aretaeus's concept and viewed
the sexual organs as "animals within the animal." But it was the irrepressible wanderlust of the womb that achieved the most remarkable notoriety in the history of medicine. Belief in this egregious
notion persisted in one form or another in medical thinking until
at least the 17th century.

In Hippocratic medicine, the wanderings of the womb are not
entirely the erratic impulses of a wild beast. They are determined
by a peculiar sensitivity of the uterus to the variations of temperature and humidity in its environment. Dry and cold as this quin-
tessentially feminine viscus is, it is only natural that it should seek
after warmth and humidity. Both could be supplied by the liver,
but above all they are furnished by semen. However, semen is not
always available to the womb, and this organ, in its efforts to find
warmth and to avoid excessive dehydration, undergoes very wide
and violent displacements. Its lurches, so to speak, may interfere
with the respiratory airway, and when that happens, the patient
suffers a dreadful crisis characterized by asphyxia—a hysteric crisis. Through the 18th century and the early 19th, medical texts still
spoke of "the suffocation of the *mother*" (a synonym of the uterus),
a symptom that was among the most feared manifestations of hys-
teria—the word, after all, comes from the Greek ὑστέρα, womb.

Thus, Hippocratic medicine hit upon the singular notion of an organ endowed with spontaneous mobility yet ruled by certain natural laws. This medical system also maintained that health could be restored only if the displaced uterus were brought back to its normal location. The outrageous measures to which ancient physicians resorted in order to restore a rebellious womb to its normal place have been commented on by numerous authors.

But if the womb was an animal, what sort of animal was it? When I was a medical student, I learned that the uterine cervix (the part of the uterus that protrudes into the vagina, and which may be seen with the aid of the speculum; in other words, the "gynecologist's view" of the womb) presents an opening whose common technical name, in countries of Latin-derived language, is "tench's muzzle" (in Spanish, *hocico de tenca*). I confess that for some time I did not know what a tench was. It is, as I found out, a freshwater fish of the carp family (scientific name *Tinca tinca*) that can measure between 7 and 14 inches in length and weigh up to four and one-half pounds. The tench is noted for its ability to survive for some time outside of its watery environment and is highly valued as a table fish. Is the uterus then to be likened to a fish? Not quite. A revered European textbook of anatomy first published in the 19th century states:

> The intravaginal segment [of the cervix uteri] is shaped like a cone whose vertex, directed downward, appears truncated and rounded; in some cases this appearance may be exaggerated (cervix in *mole's muzzle* of Sims; cervix in *tapir's muzzle* of Ricord) and become a cause of infertility.[10]

The uterus a mole? A tapir? A table fish? On a more prosaic plane, the cervix uteri, from the gynecologist's vantage point, appears as a rounded structure with a hole in the center; it resembles nothing so much as a doughnut. Natalie Angier, in her delightful book on feminine biomedicine, *Woman: An Intimate Geography*, says that a gynecologist she met confessed that doing pelvic examinations made her hungry. The doctor wasn't trying to be facetious or racy, "she just liked doughnuts."[11]

The hoariest uterine similes, however, have been marine. An admirably erudite study of the talismans or amulets used by women of the classical Greco-Roman period to propitiate a normal childbirth shows that the uterus was first represented as a cupping vessel, but gradually this iconographic symbolism changed into an octopus.[12] As a marine animal, the octopus, like the uterus, can thrive only in a well-hydrated environment; it cannot stand desiccation. Its long tentacles enable it to move in any direction, any time that it feels the need to do so. Moreover, the consistency of the uterine cervix, as we have seen, was compared by Soranus to that of the head of an octopus. Galen deepened the resemblance by proposing the existence of suckers in the uterine inner surface, called "cotyledons" (Greek, *kotyledon*, a cup-shaped depression), just like those present in the tentacles of an octopus. Presumably, by means of these formations, the placenta would adhere firmly to the uterine walls. It may be that Galen extrapolated to the human species observations made on the uterus of some ruminants, which may actually have depressions vaguely evocative of suckers. The term *cotyledons* was preserved in medicine to designate the lobes separated by fissures that can be seen on the maternal surface of the placenta.

Greco-Roman medicine recommended octopus in the diet of women suffering from infertility. Eating octopus was also supposed to help parturient women to more speedily eliminate the *lochia* (discharge from the uterus and vagina that follows after delivery).[13] In ancient Athens, a family feast called *amphidromia* (ἀμφιδρόμια) was celebrated shortly after the birth of a child. During the ceremony, the child received consecration and a name. Gifts were brought to the mother during this festivity; octopus to be consumed as food was among the traditional presents.

The zoomorphism of the uterus does not finish here. An erudite Swiss antiquarian, Véronique Dasen, informs us that in Egyptian amulets, Khepri, the scarabee-god that propitiates an uneventful childbirth, appears sometimes in close proximity to the figure that represents the uterus and sometimes takes the place of the uterus itself[14] (the uterus as divine insect!). She also notes a transition between the stylized iconography of the octopus—a circle with radial lines or tentacles extending from its surface—and the representation of the head of Medusa, from whose rounded head emanate serpents instead of hairs. The choice of Medusa, a deadly, frightening monster, as a symbol of the uterus seems surprising at first, but as Dasen points out, there exists a long tradition of anthropomorphic comparisons to this organ. The uterus, like the human head, has a neck (cervix) continuous with the body (fundus), a "mouth" (Greek *stoma*) that leads to its interior, and "lips," as the edges of this mouth are still referred to in modern medicine.

It hardly needs to be said that the use of Medusa as a representation of the uterus betrays complex feelings of fascination mixed with fright, which have endured in the minds of men. Medusa is

the face of a being that it is "impossible to see"—a prodigious, preternatural presence at one time "terrible to look at" and "marvelous
to behold," as ancient Greek writers called her.[15] For she could be
revolting or attractive, terrifying or grotesque, and worthy of being
derided. On the one hand, Medusa is horror personified: gazing
at her causes a lethal shock; her face is the black sun of death, a
sight that can be endured only indirectly, as a reflection in a mirror. Carved on the warriors' shields, the semblance of her visage
preserves a deadly efficacy: it emits the rays of terror that dis-
hearten and subdue the enemy. On the other hand, another tradition regards her as uncannily beautiful. The Roman poet Ovid, in
book IV of his *Metamorphoses*, depicts her as "once renowned for
her loveliness," so that she evokes the envy of Athena, who trans-
forms her luscious head of hair into a bunch of writhing serpents.
Pausanias, the Greek historian, gives a different account, but one
in which her outstanding beauty is the cause of her decapitation.
Medusa leads the Libyans against Perseus, one of the great heroes
of Greek mythology, and, while encamped one night, she is perfidi-
ously assassinated. Perseus admires her beauty, even in death. He
cuts off her head—not as an act of murderous cruelty but in order
not to have to part from her splendid visage and to show its sovereign perfection to his compatriots, the Greeks.[16]

Menses

According to one interpretation of the myth, the blood gushing
forth from Medusa's decapitation is the blood of menstruation.
This physiologic phenomenon adds one more layer of mystery to
the enigma of the womb. Aristotle wrote in his treatise *On Dreams*

that women who gaze at their own image in a mirror while menstruating leave a stain on the mirror.[17] The Greeks believed that the eyes emit something particulate that can move the air before it. But the eyes, like the rest of the woman's organs, were profoundly modified by changes in the blood induced by menstruation. Something in the person of the menstruating woman flowed out, struck the polished metallic surface of the mirror, and left on it an opaque, bloodshot mark that persisted after the woman had gone away; it was like a bloody halo that could not be wiped off.

It was no coincidence that the ancients thought there was also something in that mysterious organ, the uterus, that imparted to the entire person of the woman one knows not what darksome properties in recurrent cycles. For this something, which flowed out with the menses, was generally believed to be harmful: it could sour the wine, impede the rising of leavened bread, blunt the edge of a knife, make fruits fall, rust iron and bronze, and exert countless other undesirable effects. To believe Pliny, dogs who tasted it were driven mad, and their bites became infected by an incurable poison. Still more: "even that tiny creature the ant is said to be sensitive to it and throws away grains of corn that taste of it and does not touch them again."[18]

Since biblical times, all manner of stigmas and prohibitions were foisted upon menstruating women, which better public education and the abolition of ancestral superstitions have not succeeded in totally expunging. Behind all these practices and interdictions is the fanciful notion that menstruation is a way of eliminating or expelling something unhealthy, unclean, or undesirable.

Awareness of the uterus first comes to women during puberty in the form of bleeding. Considering the ancestral, universal imagery of blood, this is a jolting experience. The idea of a wound, injury, or disease of the internal organs is difficult to avoid. Blood is life, and blood flowing out gives the impression that life is escaping. The consequences to the female's psyche are always troubling. Even if the young girl is fortunate enough to have prudent and well-informed parents or custodians whose good advice will spare her worse future miseries, the sense of fear, and perhaps shame, often marks the onset of menses.

Of the massive amount of writings devoted to this theme, perhaps none is as poignant and thoughtful as Simone de Beauvoir's landmark study, *The Second Sex*. This superb work is now more than a half century old. Feminist intellectuals worldwide have abundantly commented on its major theses, expanded its observations, and strengthened—and on occasion disputed—its major arguments. I certainly have no pretension to add to the deluge of commentary incited by that precedent-setting book, except to say that neither this avalanche of enlightened discourse, nor a greater openness of society, has abolished the widespread irrationality that surrounds the physiologic monthly bleeding. All too often, the young girl confronts the onset of menses with unrelieved anxiety. She has to contend, month by month, with the need to take certain precautions, certain manners of dress. The famous Italian criminologist Cesare Lombroso (1836–1909) suggested that the very word used for sexual modesty in Italian, *pudore* (Spanish *pudor*, French *pudeur*), comes from the Latin noun *putor* (verb *putere*), meaning bad smell or stink, suggesting that the origin of the sense of shame in women was associated with the need they perceived to suppress the bad smell associated with the menstrual flow. And he noted that this regularly repeated practice, by inuring women to dissimulation and deception, contributed to make the feminine character deceitful or disingenuous.[19]

The truth is that by this physiologic phenomenon, the young girl enters a new state, and she cannot avoid it: she is carried forcefully downstream in the inexorable current of biologic life; her life is thence defined by a "before" and "after." Before, she may have confusedly suspected the existence of a burdensome and ineluctable destiny of the female condition. After, she realizes that this obscure threat is actually ensconced inside her own abdomen.

In a grandiloquent style, author and social critic Camille Paglia invokes again the marine imagery of the uterus in connection with the menses: "Every month, it is woman's fate to face the abyss of time and being, the abyss which is herself."[20] Woman is the "abyss," in the sense that her life-giving powers take origin from the primeval, dark subterranean domain which is earth's engendering stratum: that part of the world where the seeds germinate, where roots draw nutriment, and where flowers and trees grow from. But woman relates to still another abyss: woman is the ocean, and if menstruation is associated with ideas of revulsion and shame, Paglia tells us, it is not on account of the blood flowing out but because of "the albumen in the blood, the uterine shreds, placental jellyfish of the female sea."[21]

Paglia's colorful wording and pithy marine metaphors are not new: the like expressions may be found in virtually the entire world's literatures. Scholars who have researched archetypal ideas of the feminine know that these are often linked to aquatic-oceanic imagery. All of which did not impede Natalie Angier from coming up with a mischievous quip: "Placental jellyfish? [. . .] this woman needs to be confined to an aquarium."[22]

Considering the problems associated with menstruation, might it not be better to suppress it altogether? This question, which may seem surprising, was posed in all earnestness by modern medicine. So it is that scientists at pharmaceutical firms have worked to find a solution, and their efforts were rewarded. In May 2007, the U.S. Food and Drug Administration approved the commercialization of a birth control pill, Lybrel, from Wyeth Pharmaceuticals. This medicament not only prevents pregnancy but also eliminates menses: the women who take it will not menstruate.

As reported in an editorial of the *New York Times*, a presentation of this drug to investors and health professionals was bolstered by quoting published scientific evidence of the negative aspects of menstruation.[23] Nor is this surprising: at one time or another, studies have shown, presumably with all the impartiality of science, that menstruating women report more sick days while gainfully employed, contributing to drive up the absentee rate and thus damage the economy; that their tendency to use dark clothes on certain "critical" days redounds to the detriment of the clothing industry; and that the fact that many tend to feel sick for several days month by month, repeatedly throughout the best years of life, is an indication that they are unfit for any activity demanding sustained mental and physical effort. Needless to say, these arguments have been used to deny women access to activities and professions long considered to be the exclusive prerogative of males. Gender discrimination not uncommonly adopted the guise of chivalrous protectionism: women were simply "too weak" and had to be prevented from harming themselves.

However, the upright gentlemen who so wished to protect women from harm were never known to initiate a crusade to defend farm girls, maids, servants, and sundry other females engaged in strenuous occupations that demanded muscular effort disproportionate to their strength. As stated in the aforementioned editorial, allegedly unbiased scientific arguments demonstrating the socially harmful effects of woman's physiology have been used in the past and tend to reappear according to social and cultural determinants that have nothing to do with science. Thus, during World War II, when women were needed at the factories, any complaints of not feeling well because of menses were dismissed as soppy self-coddling. Women were told that there was abundant scientific evidence that they were perfectly fit during periods; these were perfectly natural; why, even during bleeding, there was no cause to make a fuss. Then, after the war was over and women were no longer needed at the workplace, a fresh new wave of studies appeared showing that the work environment was harmful to them, that their children needed them at home, and that they were less efficient workers than men. It is perhaps significant that the affliction known as "premenstrual syndrome" first appeared in 1953, coinciding with the pressures that compelled women to quit their jobs and stay at home.

But if having a functional uterus is a bother, having one that ceases to function is no less a one. (In connection with this organ, it seems, women simply cannot win!) The menopausal syndromes associated with a womb that ceases to respond to hormonal stimuli have generated innumerable medical writings and a commensurate amount of sociologic commentary. Menopause has also given rise to surgical abuse, for there is evidence that at this phase of life, many uteruses are removed without valid medical indication. I will forgo developing this topic here, as its appropriate development would lengthen this chapter unnecessarily. But I cannot refrain from remarking that the treatment of the uterus by the medical profession is emblematic of medicine's current excess.

Medicine in our time has failed to recognize its own boundaries. Every phase of our lives must come under medical superintendence: birth, growth, development, adolescence, senescence, and death are, to use a current term, being "medicalized." A uterus that bleeds monthly is subject to pharmacological suppression under questionable premises, just as a uterus that stops bleeding due to age is subject to surgical extirpation, often for reasons no less questionable.

When will medicine recognize its limits? The "hyperactive" need sedation; the depressed need stimulants; the short, growth hormone; the overweight, appetite suppressants; the lean, nutritional supplements; and for every difficult pass in life there exists an ad hoc pharmacologic lenitive. We are witnessing what Jules Romains (1885–1972), French author and playwright, presciently depicted in his satirical play *Knock or the Triumph of Medicine* (1923): every person in the world, without exception, has "something" that must be treated, or as a physician says in that play, "healthy individuals are sick patients in ignorance [of their condition]."

Womb as Tomb

The idea of woman has been tinged historically with the deep neurotic fear that invariably attaches to all the great unknowns: the
deep, the immensity of the ocean, the limitless space, darkness, or
death. And so it was that woman was decked with a mythology
that answered to the troubling emotions elicited by the unknown.
She was mysterious, like dark night; unfathomable, like space; in-
satiable, like the sea; fertile, like mother earth; at once alluring and
deadly, like the abyss. The giver of life, but also the incarnation
of death—Medusa, the Fates, the Furies, and Death itself were
commonly represented as female—she was womb and tomb at the
same time: womb and tomb, and the two inextricably joined, indis-
tinguishable from each other.

Yet the life-death antinomy that, conditioned by education,
we tend to accept, is nowhere better exposed as spurious than in
the menstrual cycle. We have been taught to welcome life as the
greatest good and, therefore, to fear death as the utmost evil; life is
seen as all plenitude and affirmative energy; death, as all rarefaction
and negativity. But biology, and in particular menstrual physiology, reminds us that this trenchant, Manichean opposition is an
artificial construct; that life and death are coextensive with each
other, complementary to each other, and, in a profound sense, the
same thing. To clarify this idea, we must take a closer look at the
menstrual cycle.

During the first part of the cycle, the endometrium—the lining of the uterine cavity—proliferates and progressively swells in
preparation for the embryo's implantation. If fertilization does not
occur, the endometrium literally dies, and the dead cells, Paglia's

"uterine shreds," are expelled to the outside in the monthly, bloody discharge. Death takes place that a fresh bed may be prepared for a new life to nestle in. But is that all? Only recently biologists began to wonder whether this simple enunciate constitutes the whole story, and, as always in biology, the truth appears to be much more complex than believed at first. Menstruation very likely constitutes the culmination of a fine process of evolutionary adaptation of the human species. Therefore, as a physiologic process, its significance is bound to be multifaceted.

One controversial hypothesis proposed that the periodic shedding of the endometrial mucosa may protect against infections.[24] A ripe, swollen endometrium, full of nutrients and ready to harbor the embryo, must look like a tempting Shangri-la to the bacterial populations that swarm in the lower segments of the female reproductive system. But bacterial invasion and colonization of the uterine cavity—the precious shop of nature—are things that the woman's body must avoid at all costs. Imagine the hardy bacterial masses, allured by the sight of the Promised Land, ready to climb up and colonize the fertile endometrial plains that offer themselves in the distance. Imagine, next, how these microbial pioneers, after eluding mucus barriers and countless other perils, are ready to cross the straits of the cervix uteri, when lo! an abrupt, massive landslide takes place and sweeps away the would-be settlers, who tumble down to extinction amidst torrents of blood and endometrial shreds.

In another hypothesis, the endometrium dies and sheds because to be maintained in a state of readiness for embryo implantation would be far too costly in terms of energy.[25] A uterus about to receive the fertilized egg is not merely rigging itself in a swollen, "succulent" inner lining. It is also sending and receiving innumerable signals, many of a hormonal nature, others still unknown or incompletely understood, by means of which the entire female body readies itself for the extraordinary task of procreation. As a ship's crew busies itself fitting sails, braces, and stays to the masts and spars when about to put to sea, so the uterine tissues, before setting off on the voyage of engendering, must sound the general alarm of the impending task. Muscle cells prepare to stretch and divide; solid materials to mollify; blood vessels to grow; breast cells to proliferate and secrete; and the crisscrossing messages reach near and distant organs of the mother-to-be. The woman's metabolism is said to be raised as much as 7 percent above normal. Clearly, to keep this keen state of diligent wariness forever would be impractical, wasteful of energy, and outright harmful. Nature then does what is called for: she induces the collective suicide, the massive death of all the "primed" endometrial cells, and a new cycle starts over.

Massive death-life cycles take place everywhere in our body; millions of cells become effete, die, and are replaced, but we remain blissfully unaware of this occurrence because this cellular holocaust courses in silence. Human granulocytes (a type of white blood cell) die and are replaced at the amazing rate of 1.3 million per second.[26] The cells of the superficial layers of the skin are constantly dying, flaking off, and being renewed, at such a speed that it may be truthfully said that we molt faster than snakes. Cell death and renewal are no less formidable in the gastrointestinal tract. Many cells carry within themselves the genetic plan that impels them to self-destruction by a specific form of death—apoptosis is the technical term—which has been likened to a "cell's suicide."

Embryo-fetal development is the most staggering example conceivable of growth and proliferation: an invisible, microscopic living particle becomes a whole 2,500- to 3,000-gram human infant in barely nine months! Without going beyond the modest limits of human life, here we touch on the portentous. Jean Rostand was right to say that in order to become frightened, man has no need to gaze into the depths of Blaise Pascal's infinities: it suffices him to look into himself. One would expect that during the explosive process of human generation, the plenitude of life should be perfect, complete, and unbroken. Yet it is at this time that death is ubiquitous and most prevalent. If the embryo's organs are to adopt their final shape, millions of cells have to die. The usual example given is the formation of the limbs: when first formed in the embryo, they are finlike appendages or buds that look like solid paddles; for fingers to appear, solid tissue has to be removed, as when a sculptor chisels out a block of marble in order to shape the fingers of a statue's hand. If some tissue were not removed, our hands would end up webbed, like duck's feet. The excised tissue dies by apoptosis. Nor is organ shaping (morphogenesis) the only instance of wholesale cellular suicide in the embryo. In the production of some organ systems, notably the kidneys, the embryo forms "preliminary" organs destined to disappear. These are organs that, as the embryo grows, become obsolete and insufficient to satisfy the enhanced physiological demands. At that point, the millions of cells that make up these fully formed precursor organs oblige the host by killing themselves.

Thus, from our earliest beginnings and throughout our entire lives, life and death are both equally in attendance inside our bodies. But of this binary presence, we know nothing. Menstruation is the only conspicuous token of those cycles of life and death regularly occurring inside the organism, and only the female half of humanity receives a monthly reminder that "in the midst of life we are in death." Apoptosis, a distinctive form of cell death (for cells indulge different styles of self-annihilation), became known only in the 1970s. Present-day biology views apoptosis as an equal and opposite force to mitosis, the cell's division. Billions of our cells succumb throughout our lives. If they did not, the consequences would be terrible: imagine our epidermis thickening gradually to a grotesque degree, vastly surpassing that of a rhinoceros; imagine organs and bodily appendages growing disorderly into such awful deformities as would make life's continuance impossible; imagine new and appalling forms of pathology brought about by the persistence and proliferation of cellular systems that normally disappear during our lives. All because the life of normal cells would not be counterbalanced by their necessary demise. As the eminent pathologists Guido Majno and Isabelle Joris put it, "*these normal cycles of cell life and death cannot be interrupted without threatening the survival of the individual* [their italics]."[27]

Soberly considered, the monthly visible, obtrusive, bloody reminder of recurrent death cycles in the living female body should make us reconsider the traditional symbolism of life and death. For death is not the awful, discarnate skull that we discover late, after many years, when the superficial layers of the organism have been slowly and relentlessly peeled away. Death is not like a second nature that would exist only in a latent state behind our external appearance, to become an unwanted material presence at the end of life's journey. Neither is death a strange menace that lies deeply concealed at the bottom of all depths, ready to pounce on us, the living, when we least expect it. No, it is not hidden and subterranean but out in the light of immediate facts; coexistent and coeval with life and indispensable for life's continuance. Biology conclusively proves that without the simultaneous or alternating cycles of life and death, the very *survival of the individual* would be impossible. So it is that the best life-death symbolism ought not to invoke two antagonistic and mutually counteractive principles but use instead images that represent two aspects of the same thing. The trite example is the obverse and reverse of the same coin, neither of which may be destroyed without invalidating the whole. Majno and Joris add the striking suggestiveness of an ancient Aztec sculpture kept at the National Museum of Anthropology in Mexico City, Mexico: viewed from the front, it represents a living jaguar, but viewed from the back, it shows the beast's skeleton.[28]

If only we could view life and death by the light of the biologic knowledge that our species has so tenaciously pursued and so painstakingly conquered, the terrors of death would lose their bite, and much existential despair and anxiety would seem groundless. But, alas, our lot is not to see the world through the diaphanous lenses of knowledge-*cum*-reason, but through a thick layer of human hopes, desires, yearnings, fears, expectations, ambitions, hungers, fancies, faiths, blind beliefs, and plain irrationality. The kind of emotional overlay that makes us see what we wish to see, not what is in front of us. Hence the ambivalence toward menstruation.

Regarded by the light of reason, its life-death cellular cycles are nothing but a physiologic process necessary for the continuation of life. But from a strictly human perspective, these cycles embody a mighty clash that we cannot look upon with indifference. For they seem to us to enact a fight between the forces that would annihilate us—which we passionately refuse—and those that affirm life and promise us a new beginning, a new dawn, a second birth.

No writer has treated the ambivalent significance of uterine bleeding with greater poignancy than Thomas Mann in his troubling novella *Die Betrogene* (*The Deceived One*). [29] In it, a fiftyish, gray-haired German widow, Frau Rosalie von Tümmler, experiences a strong erotic attraction for Ken Keaton, an American young man more than 20 years her junior, who is her teenage daughter's English language teacher.

First published in the United States in the 1950s, the novella was unfavorably received. The puritanical America of those years was bothered by the strong, unmistakable erotic tone of the feelings described by the writer in a middle-class European matron. The prevailing conventional morality adjudicated this inadmissible; some called it plainly "disgusting." Yet the development of the woman's feelings is masterfully chronicled. This brief book is one of the few narratives authored by a male writer and convincingly told from the female point of view. Tolstoy comes to mind, as being one of those exceptional writers able to cast off the male personality and tell a story with a distinctly feminine sensibility, as if by some thaumaturgic transformation he had been able to appropriate a woman's heart and mind. Very few others have accomplished this extraordinary feat.

In Thomas Mann's story, the middle-aged woman loves as she had never loved before and is stirred to the very root of her being by desire. She is a decent person, and not exempt of a certain sense of shame when her passion flares up. Then she begins to have uterine bleeding, and this makes her very happy. She was already menopausal, but the resumption of the bloody discharge is exhilarating for her. Nature, she thinks, has restored "her physical womanhood" at the prompting of the emotions that the young man has stirred in her. She thought her body was past the time of biologic generation, when lo! there comes what looks like a sign of fecundity and thus a sign of her corporeal receptivity to the male embrace.

This singular development seems to her perfectly understandable. Love has the power to mobilize the deepest biologic resources. Menopause, she thinks, has been made to reverse its course. Love rekindles a body that was dormant but not completely exhausted. For love sets in motion the very principles that oppose death and affirm that the end is not yet reached: germination, fructification, burgeoning, and efflorescence—all are awakened. She thought that her body had withered? Was she beginning to somber in a foretaste of death? Well, now she menstruates again! Love has given her a second chance, set her upon a new departure. Erotic love is the warmth that defrosts a life that seemed frozen, fixed, and without future. Now, she believes in her exultation, there is a future for her.

Buoyed by the ardency of her passion, full of a sense that the flow of her life, until then jammed, has been unlocked and opened once again to numberless unrealized possibilities, she yields to the solicitations of her heart and arranges an outing to Holterhof Castle with the young man and her children. There she manages to find a few moments alone with her beloved and reveals her love to him. This confession takes place in the moldy and decaying passages of the old castle (a deliberate symbol of the body's ineluctable aging and decay?). It is not a fit place for the consummation she yearned after. It was in gentle nature, fanned by a soft breeze "amidst the sweet perfume of jasmines and alders" that she dreamed it should be, "not in this grave!" She promises that she will come to him in his room the next morning, perhaps that same evening.

But Frau von Tümmler does not go to the planned tryst. The next morning finds her indisposed: the uterine bleeding has suddenly become alarmingly profuse. She is taken to the hospital, and a medical examination yields a definite diagnosis. The reason for the bleeding was not, as she erroneously believed, a resumption of menstruation after the onset of menopause, but a very different condition: a malignant tumor of the uterus. She was deceived. She took for a promise of new life what was, in reality, a harbinger of death.

The cancer is too far advanced. The doctors attempt a surgical removal of the tumor, but under the strong, white light of the operating room lamps, it becomes clear that the spread of the cancer is too extensive to hope for even a temporary improvement: the malignancy has become implanted in multiple foci in the peritoneum, all the lymph nodes are massively involved by carcinoma, and there are metastases in the liver.

As Rosalie von Tümmler lies dying, she has no regrets, she utters no words of bitterness. She does not consider herself deceived.

Nature, she tells her daughter, is not a defrauder; there is no ill will or maliciousness in her actions. True, she laments having to leave the world, and life with its spring. "But how should there be a spring without death? Indeed, death is a great instrument of life." And she adds that, in her case, death presented itself "in the guise of resurrection, of the joy of love"—and *that*, she concludes with unwavering finality, was not deceit, "not a lie, but goodness and mercy."

Part II: Male

On Erectile Tissue and Some of Its Misfortunes

De Secretis Mulierum ("On the Secrets of Women") was the title of a highly regarded written work initially attributed to the erudite 13th-century Dominican monk and naturalist Albertus Magnus, although it was probably authored by one of his followers. It is not the only medieval composition that joined the idea of secrecy to the constitution of women: throughout the 14th and 15th centuries, other writings continued to appear with identical or similar titles—whether in Latin, intended for the learned, or in the vernacular, for a wider public—all affirming that secrecy is consubstantial to women.[30] Two things were meant by this expression: first, that there was a type of knowledge open only to women, since men were traditionally excluded from attending childbirths and remained woefully ignorant of the most elementary facts of female anatomy and physiology, not to mention gynecological diseases; and second, that the organs responsible for female sexuality were, on the main, utterly hidden and frustratingly inaccessible. In other words, "secret."

Placed deep in the pelvic cavity, the chief components of the female reproductive apparatus may be said to have developed, literally as well as figuratively, in the shade. It is quite otherwise with the male sexual organs, which are all exteriority and conspicuousness. Looking at the male body, it is difficult to suppress the thought that the genital apparatus was an add-on, a belated appending; as if a demiurge had been in charge of fashioning the male human body, and, when getting ready to proudly declare his task finished, while standing back to better contemplate his masterpiece, had suddenly smacked his own forehead with the palm of his hand and exclaimed, "Dear me! I forgot!" upon realizing that he had given no thought to the genital system. We may further imagine that, to remedy this oversight, he had hurriedly fashioned the organs that he deemed appropriate to the generative function and, with a look of sheepish contrition and self-reproach, simply tacked them onto the outside of his finished creature.

But this consideration inevitably leads us to question the Freudian concept of "penis envy," according to which the female of the human species, at a very early age, realizes the physical difference that exists between the sexes, and experiences her own condition as a deficiency, as a lack, or, in Freudian terms, as a castration. The concept of penis envy occupied a very prominent place in psychiatric thought for several generations. In this view, envy leads to self-loathing: realizing that she lacks an organ which she cannot have, the female identifies herself as the lesser of the two participants in the extremely important sphere of sexual life, and seeks to compensate for this deficiency by tortuous mental schemes of substitution. Yet Freud never satisfactorily explained why the infantile female mind must experience the difference as a deficiency, let alone a castration.

In other words, what evidence did he have to postulate the mentioned reaction? Why would a little girl automatically assign her own condition to an inferior rank in comparison to the male's, instead of underrating the male structure, marked as it is by what seems an awkward, belated addition? Why must she be self-derogatory, when in fact she might have disparaged the male, contrasting the purity of line proper to the female body to what conceivably could be called, in the male, an anti-aesthetic excrescence? The truth is that Freud had little objective evidence to support his hypothesis. In recent times, psychiatrists and intellectuals in various disciplines have suspected the presence of sheer male prejudice as the chief stay of his theorizing. And would it not be equally tenable to invert the terms and to propose that the male is envious of the female's ability to procreate? There is abundant historical evidence that men have nurtured a jealousy for what nature begrudged them. Why not hypothesize a male envy of the uterus rather than a female envy of the penis? But these criticisms have been eloquently formulated by several scholars. Here it is not our intention to add to this mass of commentary, and we return to our coarser approach to human corporeality.

The penis, the anatomical part which is considered emblematic of maleness, is a roughly cylindrical structure with a bulbous cap, or glans, arising in front of, and beneath, the pubis. It is all exterior, yet it too has an inside. But to observe it, it is necessary to perform a series of transverse sections, as if one were cutting a sausage into discoid slices. (Horror! The mere thought of this strikes unendurable dread in the heart of males.) It then becomes apparent that the penile cylinder is not single-bodied but is actually composed of two fleshy cords that originate back in the perineum, then come together, and run closely apposed to each other along the length of the penile shaft, which is thus traditionally compared to a two-barreled gun. These are the corpora cavernosa, cigar-shaped, spongy formations appropriately named on account of the multitude of interconnecting, labyrinthine spaces, or cavities, which thoroughly pervade their substance. Although these structures are paired and a fibrous septum marks the zone at which the two are joined, this dividing wall is actually incomplete, containing many fenestrations that allow the flow of blood between them.[31] Functionally, the two sections behave as one: when blood flows into them, the blood pressure is the same in both.

At the undersurface of the corpora cavernosa, as a result of the two parallel cylindrical cords adjoining each other, a furrow is formed where lodges a third cylindrical structure, albeit of much narrower caliber than the other two, and endowed with less spongy tissue. It is the corpus spongiosum, this one single, which houses and protects the urethra, the tube through which urine and semen are expelled. At its distal tip, the corpus spongiosum is capped by the glans, a sort of helmet, as it were, of the male organ.

It must be owned that the demiurge who showed himself improvident in belatedly attaching the sexual organs to the outside of the male human creature amply made up for this lack of foresight by crafting an instrument that is a marvel of bioengineering.

The way its various constitutive elements are disposed has right-fully been a subject of wonder among physiologists and medical scientists. The intended goal is to transform a flaccid organ, sustained by a low volume of blood at low pressure, into an effective copulatory device. This is achieved by converting it into a high-pressure, high-volume biologic system, and to this effect, each component piece is exquisitely designed, crafted, regulated, and harmonized with the rest.

In the technical jargon of experts in biomechanics, "Penises are variable-volume hydrostatic skeletons."[32] From a purely physical perspective, the axial array of orthogonal collagen fibers, cleverly arranged at 0 degrees and 90 degrees to the long axis, confers to this organ a firm, erect posture that resists bending. Moreover, the fibers are disposed so as to change from the flaccid to the distended state in a most efficient manner. From a biologic standpoint, the precision of every step in the process of changing its shape could not be more astounding. Nervous and hormonal stimuli bring messages that open up arteries and relax muscle fibers, thus allowing the influx of arterial blood. The spongelike corpora cavernosa swell upon being suffused with blood. The constituent cells release chemicals that enhance their respective functions and inhibit the contrary effects. The veins are so disposed that they become compressed against the tough fibrous sheath that surrounds the penile shaft, limiting the egress of the blood and thereby ensuring the rigidity of the organ. Suffice it to say that an erection exemplifies the consummate perfection that went into penile design; its admirable physiologic precision, still incompletely understood, is well served by a uniquely suited structure.

I first learned about the microscopic constitution of the corpora cavernosa as a medical student. I was fortunate to have assuaged my curiosity in a textbook written with flair and a charming sense of humor—qualities that, sadly, remain extremely rare in medical textbooks. If my memory serves me right, it was the Spanish-language translation of the first (probably pirate) edition of Emmerich von Ham's textbook of histology, today unobtainable. Here was described the marvel of beauty and organization displayed in the microscopic anatomy of the corpora cavernosa. A multitude of densely crowded, intercommunicating chambers lined by endothelial cells, partitioned by delicate septa, coursed by tenuous nerve fibrils, embellished by collagen, elastic fibers, and muscle cells, the whole ensheathed in a tough, white capsule (albuginea)—all this and more the histologist may see in glorious, multicolored microscopic preparations.

The textbook then informed us that this cellular arrangement constitutes the so-called erectile tissue and added the curious detail that this kind of tissue exists only in two places: the corpora cavernosa of the penis (or its female counterpart, the clitoris), and the nose. Indeed, tissue with the described characteristics happens to be present deep in the nasal cavity, in the soft parts that cover the lower turbinate bone (one of several bony plates extending from front to back on the lateral wall of the nasal cavity, on both sides). Recent research shows that erectile tissue exists in the nasal septum and upper turbinate bone as well.[33] That its presence should be confined to the nose and the genital area raises a number of intriguing questions. Why here? And why in anatomic sites so distant from each other? Does this imply some form of nasal-genital relationship? If so, what manner of rapport is this?

My textbook provided no answers to these questions, but skirted them with characteristic humor by introducing an anecdote without, alas, mentioning its source. It stated that there was once a gentleman member of the refined 18th-century French royal court who suffered ridicule due to his inability to demonstrate the expected *galanterie* toward the ladies. (In Diderot's great *Encyclopedia*, galanterie is defined as "the marked attentiveness to say to women, in a fine and delicate way, things that please them, and which give them a good opinion of themselves and of us. This art, which might serve for their improvement and consolation, is only too often used to corrupt them.") In France, 18th-century courtly manners had rendered mandatory this "art," as Diderot calls it—actually a sort of elegant flirt—for all men who wished to prosper in high social circles; but it seems that the poor chap mentioned in my histology textbook was racked with ceaseless, unstoppable sneezing every time that he approached an attractive young woman!

After my initial encounter with this questionable historical tidbit, I heard no more about the nasal erectile tissue throughout medical school or later in my practice as a pathologist. However, an ancient popular tradition exists in many countries that links the size of a man's nose to the size of his virile member and/or the magnitude of his sexual potency. Of the hoary nature of this belief we can be sure, since a physician of the early Renaissance, Laurent Joubert (1529–1528), referred to it in a book he wrote about old superstitions and folk beliefs in medicine (*Erreurs populaires et propos vulgaires touchant la médecine et le régime de santé*, Bordeaux, 1579). The same idea seems to live in the "Dance of the Noses" of the Nuremberg mastersinger, Hans Sachs (1494–1576), performed at carnival.

Outside of popular culture and folklore, however, the presence of erectile tissue in the nose seems to occupy an insignificant
place in medicine, even among specialists. Yet it was not always
so. The nasal-genital connection found a champion in doctor
Wilhelm Fliess (1858–1928), Austrian physician and close friend
and confidant of none other than Sigmund Freud. Wilhelm Fliess
owes his place in the history of medicine chiefly to his closeness
to Freud during the years of this famous man's greatest productivity, the critical time when the concepts of the unconscious and the
Oedipal complex were taking shape in his mind. Freud famously
declared that if psychoanalysis were to be credited with only the
discovery of the Oedipus complex, "that alone would give a claim to
be included among the precious new acquisitions of mankind."

Historians generally agree that Fliess exerted an important
influence upon Sigmund Freud. The illustrious founder of psychoanalysis had a high regard for Fliess's ideas and was grateful
for his support against a medical community that showed itself
hostile or impervious to his revolutionary hypotheses. However,
their friendship was not so strong as to endure the strain of their
discrepancies. Since each one was utterly persuaded of the truth
of his convictions, their differences became irreconcilable, and the
friendship eventually came to an ungracious end.

As a specialist in ear, nose, and throat diseases, Fliess was sensitive to all matters nasal. He was aware that erectile tissue is shared
by the organs of sex and olfaction. He noted that some women
bleed through the nose in synchrony with their menses or in lieu of
the same, and that bleeding may stop simultaneously in the genital
and nasal areas. He also knew that sexual arousal, like pregnancy,

is accompanied by swelling of the erectile tissues in the nasal fossa. With these flimsy and dispersed bits of evidence, and a number of abstract arguments drawn from natural history, he built his own pet theory.[34] Is it not true that olfaction plays a major role in animal sexual activity? The cosmetic industry uses the odorous secretions of sebaceous, anal, or genital glands of some mammals, such as civet cat, muskrat, deer, and beaver to prepare fragrances and perfumes. And it is generally known that ants, moths, and butterflies emit pheromones. Since it is a fact that emanations perceived by the sense of smell are powerful sexual attractants and determinants of sexual behavior in many living species, it seemed right to ask, why not in humans? The idea that there is a fundamental concordance between sexuality and nasality became a dogma in Fliess's mind.

Proceeding to examine in great detail the nasal mucosa of his patients, he convinced himself (but could it have been otherwise?) that he saw "genital spots"—that is, areas of the nasal mucosa that were particularly swollen in various pathologic states, such as migraine headaches or painful menstruation (dysmenorrhea). From here there was only one small step to conclude that the visible changes in the genital spots were the *cause* of the disorder. This step was promptly taken when he began to treat those patients by anesthetizing the culprit spots with cocaine. Need we say that he believed these patients showed improvement after the application of this therapy? Nor is there any reason to doubt that the patients must have experienced a sense of well-being after a cocaine "high," but the relief was only temporary.

Because Sigmund Freud referred many of his patients to Fliess, the two colleagues often had to treat psychological ailments.

No matter: the many symptoms of neurosis could be treated intranasally. Freud considered Fliess as his mentor in some respects and received his fanciful ideas with enthusiasm. Thus, the reciprocal relationship between nasality and sexuality was built into a dogma. Both men were convinced of the merits of their unorthodox therapeutic approach, which we may call a transnasal approach to the mind. Both belonged to a generation profoundly influenced by Darwin's theory of evolution, for this momentous scientific theory was formulated and published during their own lifetime. Soon Fliess dressed his speculation in Darwinian garb: sexuality and sense of smell, so intimately joined in the lower animals, had persisted, he thought, as an evolutionary remnant in human beings—a biologic inheritance handed down from their prehuman ancestors. It ought to be said, in fairness, that these notions were received with earnest approval by luminaries of psychiatric medicine contemporary to Freud, such as Richard von Krafft-Ebing (1840–1902) and Josef Breuer (1842–1925).

Carried away by his "discovery," Fliess dreamed of everlasting fame. A large number of symptoms affecting many bodily systems, such as palpitations, sweats, headaches, nausea, vomiting, depression, and so on, he attributed to dysfunction of the nasal-sexual axis, or else he thought they were triggered by the "nasal reflex," to use his terminology. He and Freud believed that the day would come when a baffling array of pathologic conditions would be recognized as caused by the proposed nasal etiology; then multiple disparate ailments would be conceptualized as one disease and be known the world over as "Fliess's disease." For the golden dream of many a clinician—the highest honor and crowning apotheosis, as it were, of those in the medical field—is to have their names indissolubly linked to some awful malady.

Since the cause of the illness was assumed to reside in the nasal cavity, it seemed feasible to remove it definitively. Obviously, a permanent cure was preferable to the temporary alleviation that cocaine afforded. Hence the more radical treatments to which Fliess resorted. Sigmund Freud diagnosed a woman named Dora as suffering from a "neurosis induced by masturbation," and the two good doctors concluded that this illness "could be cured" by cauterization of the nasal genital spots. Cauterization, and better yet, total ablation of the offending focus, seemed eminently rational therapies.

In 1895 Freud referred another woman with what he diagnosed as a sexuality-based neurosis to his respected colleague. Her name was Emma Eckstein. She complained of headaches, nosebleeds, and sundry manifestations that, to Freud's eye, could spring only from thwarted sexuality. Fliess performed a surgical operation consisting of the complete removal of the lower turbinate bone and adjacent tissue, in an effort to extirpate the cause of the accursed nasogenital reflex. This was the beginning of a whole string of troubles.

Following the operation, things did not go well at all. The patient had recurrent episodes of bleeding, headaches, fainting spells, swelling of the face, and sharp pain at the operative site, to which was added a persistent, fetid odor that became more noticeable as days went by. Additional consultants were brought in, but their conservative measures failed to improve the woman's condition. The hemorrhagic bouts were so severe that she became intensely pale and her pulse thready and weak. She came frighteningly close to lapsing into shock, but this could be averted by opportune conservative measures. Then a new consultant decided against conservatism and explored the surgical site. To everyone's surprise and silent consternation, he slowly pulled out a piece of gauze, over two feet long, through the patient's nostrils: it was a compressed bandage that the surgeon, Fliess, had left inside the nasal cavity. After this, Emma Eckstein made a slow recovery, except for a somewhat sunken appearance of her deboned nasal appendage. Of her neurotic symptoms, no appreciable change was perceived.

From Freud's correspondence it becomes clear that he strenuously tried to excuse Fliess's negligence.[35] He most earnestly deplored what he called "an accident" and lamented the practice of consulting on patients who live far from the treating physician, in another town, on account of the difficulty of securing the proper follow-up. But there is no denying that to leave a foreign body, such as a long segment of gauze, in the surgical site for weeks is an act of gross negligence, one that today would cost dearly for practitioners in most industrialized countries. This unfortunate happening made a profound impact on Freud's mind, as he realized when he psychoanalyzed himself, and was also the beginning of his falling out with Fliess.[36]

No medical theoretician cared to pay much attention to the nasal erectile tissue after these developments. Whatever prominence Fliess may have conferred upon it in medical discourse, it soon ebbed into the very modest role that it has had ever since. Medical men, like all those who are interested in the biology of the human being, know of its existence, but no one believes any more that important ailments affect this tissue preferentially, much less that they could originate there. It is otherwise with penile erectile tissue. Its location in the generational organ of the male endows it with an importance of the very first rank. No more needs to be added to what has already been said about the unmatched excellence of its biophysical design, except that in the very complexity of its structure lies the root of its ruin. As a tower whose bold and unprecedented architectural conception would raise it up to the clouds, higher than any other in existence, but whose weak foundation made it unsteady in proportion as it was tall, so the clever, intricate configuration of the penile erectile tissues is at the root of its vulnerability in disease.

Engorged by blood, the corpora cavernosa brook comparison to a tower, a ferule, a scepter, a staff, and many other symbols of power, domination, authority, or aggressive strength. But this arrogant symbolism of erectness is easily undone by disease and turned into its opposite: a lamentable stoop or a piteous angularity. Disease replaces the straight verticality of the erect penis with an incurved or bent organ incapable of intromission. This pitiful disorder has a name, Peyronie's disease; for here, too, we find a man whose efforts earned him the reward of being made into an eponym. In medicine, though, eponymic names are always tainted by a certain ironic ambiguity: one is at pains to know if the name designates an illustrious physician who investigated the disease, or a patient afflicted with that condition. For patients, too, have sometimes given their family name to the disease that afflicted them. By creating and sanctioning such terminology, medical professionals have tried to honor the sufferer. Although the term *Peyronie's* is in the grammatical genitive case, as indicated by its apostrophic *s*, we have no reason to believe that he *had* a bent, incurved, or otherwise deformed male organ.

Dr. La Peyronie and "His" Disease

François la Peyronie was born in Montpellier, France, on January 15, 1678. His father, Raymond la Peyronie, was a master surgeon in that city and wished to see his son elevated to a higher social stance than his own. (Recall that in those days the lot of surgeons was far inferior to that of medical doctors and not much above that of barbers, from whom they were scarcely distinguished.) To this end, he placed his child at the Jesuit College, where a solid classical education was imparted to the students. But against his father's best wishes, the young François soon showed a strong inclination to follow the surgical calling, and, thanks to an enlightened adviser, the prudent decision was taken not to oppose his preference. Because his father had earned some credit in the city, the young man was allowed to attach himself to prestigious physicians, follow them in their visits to patients, attend public and private anatomical demonstrations, and listen to some lectures by distinguished professors at the medical school. Montpellier had a long tradition in medical education and at the time was considered a sort of medical mecca in Europe.

It seems clear that the young man's early medical training was exempt from the harshness that was commonly foisted upon apprentice surgeons in the early 17th century. These were usually assigned to a master surgeon under conditions that amounted to indentured servitude. They were severely reprimanded; corrected with liberal applications of the rod; poorly fed and maintained in a chronically famished state; sent every day to the houses of men who needed shaving; and they accompanied the master in his rounds. He would entrust them with dressing of ulcers and cleaning repugnant dejections. Then they returned, fatigued, to their uncomfortable lodgings, usually an attic above the master's house, where they would sweat in the summer and clatter their teeth in the winter. There is abundant documentary evidence that these were the pains and mortifications that apprentice surgeons habitually endured, but our man, to his good fortune, escaped them. François la Peyronie grew up in the parental home, benefited from a fine medical training, and, after going through the customary tests and examinations, received his certificate of "master surgeon and barber" on February 17, 1695. He was only 17 years old when he joined a guild composed of 40 barbers in the city of Montpellier, which at the time counted about 30,000 inhabitants.[37]

His professional knowledge was commendable, his deportment was elegant, and he knew how to impress. Above all, he had the knack of dealing smoothly and persuasively with patients, which ever has been the irreplaceable, winning attribute that promotes a medical career. Thus, we see him becoming a professor at the prestigious medical school of Montpellier, treating the most exalted persons of his society, and, in 1706, becoming a member of the Royal Academy of Sciences of Montpellier. Then he gets his lucky strike. A highly placed aristocrat, the Duke de Chaulnes, afflicted with a fistula, has heard of the vaunted surgical skills of la Peyronie and summons him to Paris. We know not what kind of fistula this was; la Peyronie's biographer rests mum in this regard.

That it was a fistula-in-ano, the same distressing condition that beset King Louis XIV, we are led to suspect from the biographer's comment that "it is remarkable, according to Michelet's clever paradox, how curious a historical role was played by princely fistulas."

Our man cures the suffering duke and is rewarded with the unstinted prodigality that the powerful of those times could lavish on their favorites. A charge as surgeon in the government administration of Paris, the rank of surgeon major in the king's army, and the post of surgeon-in-chief at the Charité hospital: all these guerdons rain upon la Peyronie, who must, by royal order, make his residence in Paris. One distinction follows another: through the good offices of his many friends and his own personal talents, he is nominated a court surgeon, and in 1717 (two years after the passing of Louis XIV) receives the most coveted post, that of first surgeon of the royal person. Louis XV is only a somewhat shy, taciturn seven-year-old boy, but he is sensible to the charm of his first surgeon, who has managed to get close to him by exerting his winsome faculties upon Louis's preceptor, Abbot Fleury, and this after eluding we know not how many traps and obstacles in the traitorous corridors of the royal palace.

One more stroke of luck comes in his aid. In 1722 he has come to Reims for the fastuous ceremonies of the royal *sacre*. While there, the Duchess of Lorraine approaches him and discreetly tells him that she wishes to consult him for her husband, who suffers from—who could have guessed it?—an anal fistula! Shortly thereafter, la Peyronie performs a fistulectomy in only two minutes, "with all the speed and adroitness imaginable," according to a witness.

Next, François de la Peyronie (now we can use the particle *de*, for in the meantime he has obtained his nobility titles) gets a payment of £50,000, half in silver, half in precious gems, plus a yearly pension of 5,000 pounds; independently, the duchess gives him a diamond valued at £24,000; and, in addition, the city of Nancy, in gratitude for his having cured the revered duke, offers him 200 gold coins that bear the armorial ensign of the city on one face and that of François de la Peyronie on the other. In a modest gesture— which he could easily afford after embracing the other largesse—he accepts only a bag of silver coins. An honorarium fit to make the greediest member of today's surgical enterprises turn green!

Now our surgeon has climbed to the very top. Among his patients are the grandees of this world. The king of Poland, having fallen ill in Danzig in 1734, asks him to recommend a physician for his court. Peter the Great, czar of all Russias, comes to see him when he visits France. The king of Prussia, the elector of Cologne, and Duke Theodore of Bavaria—the list of the powerful who at one time or another become his patients is impressive. And, as it is said that there is no great man for his valet or his housekeeper, the same is true for his physician. Close to the intimacies and private weaknesses of the ruler, the physician is less prone to be overawed by the majesty of an absolute monarch: he is too familiar with the miseries and deficiencies that lurk behind the outward pomp. Thus, la Peyronie knows that the king's indiscretions have made him catch, from a young girl of a butcher's shop, what was called a "galanterie" in the coded language of courtiers, and which today would be vulgarly referred to as the clap. He treats the ruler with the best available medicaments and cures him. Obviously, this happy outcome worked wonders for his reputation as an expert in the treatment of sexually transmitted diseases—an expertise for which he was already noted, says his biographer, since his Montpellier years.

I like to imagine the elegant Monsieur de la Peyronie in his own environment. I see him in a splendid park with carefully tended lawns partitioned by gravel paths, with porphyry urns and big amphorae at the corners. There are tranquil walkways bordered by tall hedges, and bowers whose intertwined branches form umbrous canopies against the breath of summer winds. Here and there, at regular intervals, the white figure of a marble faun or a naked nymph detaches itself against the thick, green foliage. Our man, Dr. la Peyronie, is accompanied by gentlemen as careful of fashion as himself, who escort bejeweled ladies with strikingly tall, outrageously complex hairdos, and ample skirts in pink, red, yellow, or blue satin that look from afar like the corollas of flowers. They reach a monumental fountain with bronze figures of Nereids and fishes that carouse in the water, the sea nymphs spouting curved jets of water from their nipples.

What do these ladies and gentlemen talk about? A thousand nothings: they chat, they flirt, they intrigue, and the women now and then break forth in crystalline peals of laughter. But when the conversation turns to health issues, all listen to the surgeon very carefully, for every one in the group is impressed by "the nobility of his manners, the variety of his knowledge, and the politeness of his spirit," as one of his contemporaries put it. This was probably no idle flattery. For a man who was able to keep his post as first surgeon in a court chock-full of invidiousness and intrigue, where the number of internist physicians in care of the royal person (collectively named "*la Faculté du Roi*") was no less than 12, and to maintain this primacy for several decades, must have been, indeed, a person of considerable charisma and masterful diplomacy.

When the group disperses, and the men find themselves alone, they whisper to each other that the great strength of the man resides in his skills in venereology, the study and treatment of venereal diseases. They say that even in Montpellier, he was known as an expert in "this branch of the healing art," and a numerous clientele looked up to him for a remedy to the afflictions doled out by that fickle goddess, Venus. Prominent Montpellier physicians focused their attention on the treatment then in vogue for syphilis and gonorrhea, and la Peyronie made venereology his central professional interest. However, at that time, these two diseases were not yet clearly distinguished from each other, and thus the treatment, based on highly toxic mercury compounds, was administered rather indiscriminately to patients. A medical man declared that Montpellier had become "a salubrious pool for Spaniards and Italians, who came here to combat the ill that had become the scourge of Europe." What he meant was that syphilis decimated the Spaniards and the Italians, but it is well known that for them the scourge of Europe was "the French disease."

For the fact is that those polished ladies and gentlemen, so finicky in their taste and so fastidious in their dress, who passed half the morning primping themselves with narcissist titivation, were forced to spend another good part of the day pining under the torments of venereal lesions. Sophisticated, polished, and urbane as they undoubtedly were, their sexual mores were not exactly puritanical. And they paid dearly for their unrestraint, since therapies to combat venereal disease were either rudimentary or untrustworthy. A token of the prevailing situation is given by a conversation recorded by Mathieu Marais (1664–1737), advocate of the parliament of Paris and noted memorialist of the early part of the regency, during the childhood of Louis XV. Madame de Bossay was dining with the regent in the Royal Palace when she dropped this scabrous piece of gossip:

> "Monsieur the Duke has given the pox to Madame de Prie; Madame de Prie gave it to Monsieur de Livry; Monsieur de Livry gave it to his wife; his wife passed it on to la Peyronie; and la Peyronie shall cure them all."[38]

The least that can be said of such a society is that it offered a wealth of clinical material for the education of a physician interested in urology and venereal diseases. La Peyronie was such a one, and he profited from the opportunity. The disease that bears his name, he wrote, "is not rare in gentlemen of advanced age who in their youth had abandoned themselves a bit much to the vivacity of their temperament [and had contracted a venereal disease]." Yet he had enough experience to realize that in some cases the problem appeared without such antecedent; that is, in the absence of previous "pox accidents" (*accidens* [*sic*] *véroliques*). In either case, he noted areas of induration affecting the corpora cavernosa. These areas could appear as flat patches of abnormally hard tissue or as nodules protruding from the shaft of the penis "like the beads of a rosary." And he summarized many clinical observations in the following terms:

If one of these hard tumors of the corpora cavernosa is situated toward the middle of the right corpus cavernosus, the penis, instead of raising itself [during an erection] in a straight line, will describe an arch whose curvature shall be on the right side; if the hardening is on the left side, the curvature shall be equally on the side of the hardened area.

If the nodule, "rosary" or hardened area is in the part of the corpora cavernosa that faces toward the perineum, the penis will curve downward, & it will curve upward if the hardening is on the part of the corpus cavernosus that faces the pubic bones.

The curvature is always on the side of the disease: and the likely cause is as follows. The erection depends on the dilatation or swelling of the chambers of the two corpora cavernosa; if they inflate equally, no single corpus cavernosus will prevail over the other one; they will both concur equally to the same action, and the erection shall be made in a straight line; but if a hardening or drying out (*dessèchement*) in some portion of one of the two corpora cavernosa impedes the dilatation of the chambers of that portion, the corpus cavernosus will be bridled, hardened or dried out in that part; and an indentation will be formed there, which will become the center of the curvature. [39]

Today we know that the areas of "hardening" or "dryness" that the doctor was referring to are focal proliferations of fibrous tissue. La Peyronie expresses his dismay at the unresponsiveness of these lesions to the best available therapies. This makes him think that the areas of hardening are the end-stage lesions of venereal diseases, at the same title as

> scruffs (*dartres*), vague or fixed pains, & those gonorrheal
> dribblings that are refractory to mercury frictions and to
> any other [treatment] specific for pox [. . .] The frictions re-
> move the venereal virus, which, while it exists, impedes that
> these maladies be cured by the appropriate remedies. It is in
> vain that one would attack them before the virus is extinct;
> but once the virus is destroyed, these remedies can produce
> their effect, & dispel these affections.[40]

Of course, reference to a "virus," in the medical parlance of
the 18th century, denotes a poison, a toxin, or any secretion of a
living being capable of harming the organism. The word does not
have yet the contemporary meaning of a submicroscopic, DNA- or
RNA-containing living form surrounded by a protein capsule.

As to treatment, la Peyronie was forced to resort to frictions
with mercury preparations, in spite of all their disadvantages. Still,
he claimed some therapeutic successes. In one case, a 60-year-old
man had a penile area of induration that caused much pain during
erections, in addition to deviating the direction of the penile shaft
in the characteristic manner. Ejaculations were impeded by this
condition; the semen was directed inwardly to the bladder instead
of toward the outside (retrograde ejaculation); semen "could only
exit via the urethra by dribbling, after the erection had somewhat
subsided."

The patient happened to have, in addition, an old wound that
gave him pain. To treat this affliction, popular folk medicine ad-
vised bathing in some salubrious source. He went to the sulfurous,
natural warm spring of Barèges, in the High Pyrenees, at 1,250

meters of altitude. There a thermal source reputed for its alleged anti-inflammatory and antiscarring properties has been known to exist since the 14th century. The thermal waters contain a muci-laginous substance called baregine, produced by thermophillic bacteria. (The place is still much visited today by patients with various conditions, especially arthritis and other musculoskeletal diseases, who now take the salutiferous baths in spas of mod-ern construction.) La Peyronie's patient was showering with the health-giving waters of Barèges and hoping for relief from his old wound, when it occurred to him to direct the shower to his male member. After a season of such applications (we are not told how long), he noted that the induration had receded. He repeated the exposure the next season, and the results were so encouraging that he returned for a third period of treatment, after which the cure was complete: "the erections retook their ancient form, & the seed its natural ejaculation," according to the physician. Since then, la Peyronie recommended the waters of Barèges for their valuable therapeutic virtue.

La Peyronie's lasting contributions to medical science were relatively modest. Like other prominent medical men of this time, he wrote little. Yet the surgical profession is much indebted to his efforts. Not that he devised any great technical improvements or furbished important medical insights, but he caused the status of surgeons to be considerably elevated through his diplomatic abil-ity and judiciousness. One of his major accomplishments was the foundation of the French Royal Academy of Surgery, which in time became the French Society of Surgeons. Louis XV was very interested in the theory and practice of the "surgical art." Accord-ingly, la Peyronie, seriously committed to the academy, was able to increase his influence over the king. Eventually he made him realize the fundamental importance of improving the preparation of surgeons and the need to grant them the social rank to which their valuable services entitled them.

So it is that, in an official document read at Versailles on April 23, 1745, His Majesty declared, "Surgery is recognized as a learned discipline (*un art savant*), a true science which by its nature, as well as by its utility, deserves the most honorable distinctions." The same royal declaration made it mandatory for those aspiring to become surgeons to pursue preparatory studies in no way inferior in depth or comprehensiveness to those of physicians. In view of which, the royal declaration concluded in its majestic prose:

> We order that the profession of barber-surgeon being thus totally extinct, the exercise of barbering now belongs exclusively to the community of master-barbers-wigmakers-hair-dressers-bath-and-oven attendants (*baigneurs-étuviers*), all of whom shall not be permitted to exert any part of surgery."

Thus, surgery became an autonomous, respected profession, officially disassociated from that of barbers, and surgeons were elevated to the same level as physicians. Until then, the latter had exerted an invidious and oppressive domination that relegated surgeons to a subordinate place. For a long time, surgeons had been looked upon contemptuously by the university-educated physicians and were amalgamated with barbers. (Throughout the Renaissance, a duty of military surgeons in campaigns was to shave the officers.) Truly, surgeons had been considered little more than menials. It is a testimony to la Peyronie's imposing authority that no one in the powerful, influential group of physicians—who must have been seething with envy and spite—dared to protest or criticize the changes detailed in the royal declaration. The first criticisms appeared in 1749, two years after the instigator of the changes had passed away.

Appropriately, France honors his name. A statue of a sitting, dignified François de la Peyronie was placed at the entrance of the School of Medicine in his native Montpellier.

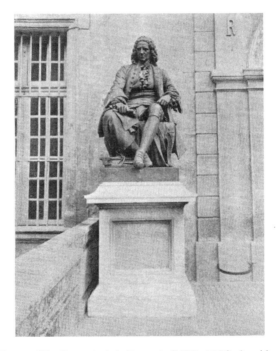

Fig. 8 Statue of Dr. François de la Peyronie (1678–1747) placed by the main door of the School of Medicine of Montpellier, France.

His portrait, kept in the French Academy of Medicine, represents him also in the sitting position, attired in sumptuous raiment indicative of his importance, wigged, and holding a beautifully bound volume, against a background of full bookshelves that signify his scholarliness and erudition.

Outside of France, however, fame did not trumpet his glory with equal resonance. Fairly comprehensive textbooks on the history of medicine fail to mention his name altogether. Well-informed physicians and medical students, upon hearing of la Peyronie, evoke the image of an elderly man whose copulatory organ has exchanged the hubris of its former straight verticality for the humiliating misery of a folded, curved, or similarly deformed condition. Perchance they think that the name Peyronie's disease alludes to some risible old fogy from legend or folklore who suffered from this affliction. And surgeons, even those who specialize in urological procedures, are usually in the dark about the man who did so much to take their trade out of its former abjection and lift it to the status of "a true science, which by its nature, as well as its utility, deserves the most honorable distinctions."

On the Representative Male Members of Representative Males

It must be because of the male organ's symbolization of life-giving energy, raw power, and authority that a morbid curiosity exists about the generational organs of men who exerted hegemony or social domination. Of this fascination, it is impossible to doubt; the evidence, both past and present, is overwhelming. And the naivety of this attitude is such that it sees power directly linked to organ size: the childish fancy is that a man who imposes his rule over his peers, who commands, influences, or controls the group, must perforce possess a copulatory organ of superior dimensions.

Hence the notorious male anxiety about size: the undersized are ridiculed, the oversized envied. The ancient Romans who attended the public baths were prone to break into spontaneous applause at the sight of a man endowed with uncommonly large penile dimensions. At least this is what Martial, the first-century Roman poet, tells us in one of his epigrams (IX, 33): *Audieris in quo, Flacce, balneo plausum, Maronis illic esse mentulam scito.* ("If you should hear, Flaccus, applause coming from the baths, you may be sure that Maron's cock is there." The Roman term for the penis, used here by the poet, is *mentula.*) Giton, a character of the Roman writer Petronius in his novel *Satyricon*, evokes the same response when he reveals his uncommonly large endowment. Straight away he finds an admirer in a Roman knight, while the crowd applauds him with "timid admiration." The well-known Roman statues of dwarfs with grotesquely large penises are thought to have been used to avert evil (apotropaic function). Perhaps even the demons of the dark underworld stopped to cheer, applaud, and extol their impressive equipment.

When Maron and Giton, obscure Roman citizens, so commanded the admiration of their contemporaries, curiosity over the genital anatomy of some great leaders seems less surprising. Yet it is striking to see, in our own times, the penises of some of history's chieftains, suzerains, or national heroes made into fetishes and highly prized collectors' items. Not since the Middle Ages, when relics from the bodies of saints were thought to preserve the attributes of holiness and the ability to work miracles, had we seen such homage and veneration directed to a bodily part sundered from its dead possessor. This fact became more intriguing to me after hearing that a professor of urology at Columbia University in New York City had managed to acquire the copulatory organ, duly preserved in fixative fluid, of no less a celebrity than France's emperor and military genius Napoléon Bonaparte (1769–1821). The matter piqued my curiosity, and I wished to find out what was behind such an allegation.

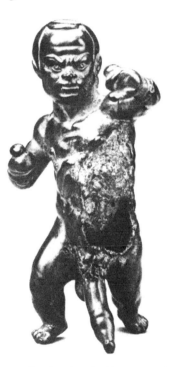

Fig. 9   Bronze statuette of boxing dwarf with grotesquely large penis. Roman, CA. A.D. 25–50.

The General and His Private

Every tourist who visits Paris knows very well that Napoléon's remains are kept in the area of the city popularly known as Les

Invalides, inside the Dome Church, or Cathedral of Saint Louis des Invalides, one of the great masterpieces in the classical style of architect Jules Hardouin-Mansart (1646–1708), built during the reign of Louis XIV. There rest the mortal despoils of the man who gave France some of its greatest glories and some of its most dolorous hours, and who left his personal mark upon the history of the Western world. He is in the company of his brothers Joseph and Jerôme, and some of his generals and marshals, all of whom are buried in lateral alcoves. In 1940 the remains of Napoléon's son François were transferred here from Vienna, where he had died in 1832.

The church at the Invalides is appropriately solemn and majestic. Directly under the glorious cupola, a circular crypt was excavated in order to house Napoléon's tomb. Two massive bronze statues guard its entrance, and 12 colossal amazon-like statues symbolizing Napoléon's military campaigns surround it, placed against the pillars that encircle the crypt. Here, at the very center of the crypt, on a floor made of tastefully inlaid color marble, rests the huge red porphyry sarcophagus upon a tall green granite base. Tourists invariably wonder about the great size of the sarcophagus, markedly disproportionate to the great man's short stature (Napoléon's autopsy report states that he measured 168 centimeters, or 5 feet, 6 inches). The guides inform them that there is not one coffin, but six, one contained inside the other and all in splendid materials: ebony, oak, tin, mahogany, and two of lead.

Would the innermost coffin enclose the body of the great leader sans the part that traditionally symbolizes physical manhood? Clearly, once the body was deposited under so formidable an enclosure, the boldest and shrewdest desecrator could not have managed to remove the said part. The dastardly deed (assuming this took place) had to be performed before the entombment. The best opportunity would have been during the handling of the corpse, especially by the physicians who performed the autopsy. Parenthetically, most French nationals know nothing about stories of the alleged postmortem castration of their national hero, and historians incline to regard the whole thing as a plainly absurd fabrication. But the last days of the emperor are exhaustively researched. As a prisoner of the English, he was heavily guarded and closely watched, and everyone close to him felt impelled to write memorials, chronicles, diaries, and sundry impressions depicting his last days. This mass of information makes it possible to speculate on how the alleged ablation might have taken place.

If anyone could have done the deed, the principal suspect is Napoléon's personal physician, Francesco Antommarchi, who performed the autopsy. Antommarchi impresses us as a quizzical, odd character. A medical eminence he certainly was not. His professional credentials are suspect. Until the age of 15, he had scarcely any formal schooling. Later he managed to go to Florence, Italy, to pursue medical studies and worked as a "prosector"—that is, an attendant in the performance of anatomical dissections at the Santa Maria Novella hospital, under Professor Giuseppe Mascagni (1755–1815), a prominent Italian anatomist.

Historians question the authenticity of his title as doctor of medicine, which he nonetheless flaunted at every opportunity. In any case, he was very young and had very limited clinical experience when he was called to serve as physician for a captive Napoléon in his exile at Saint Helena. He got the job because he was Corsican and known to the Bonaparte family. Madame *Mère*, the emperor's mother, had sworn that none but a Corsican would attend her son; and this one, a Mediterranean man to the marrow of his bones, would neither challenge the maternal authority nor trust men alien to his tribe. At length, Napoléon's mother arranged that five Corsicans be sent to keep company to her exiled son: two priests, a body servant, a cook, and the physician. But only the cook and the servant were of real service. One priest was deaf and very old; the other one was young, uncouth, and ignorant; and the physician turned out to be pretentious and incompetent.

It was Cardinal Fesch, Napoléon's maternal uncle (again, every decision was subordinate to family ties, just as in Corsica), who designated Antommarchi as physician to the exiled emperor. This was a godsend for a young physician with hardly any patients, who survived by working for a society for the diffusion of the arts and the sciences, and occupied his time by surveying the publication of a textbook of anatomy by Mascagni. Not only did the job bring him a salary of 9,000 francs, a considerable sum at the time, but it gave him the chance to name himself "physician to Napoléon," a title that he displayed ostentatiously.

He took his own sweet time before heading for Saint Helena. First he spent 40 days in Rome, then four months in London, everywhere trying to recruit subscriptions for the upcoming textbook of anatomy, and everywhere advertising himself as "physician to Napoléon." At last, he embarked for the island in the South Atlantic, where Napoléon withered under a disease that daily sapped his strength. He complained of stomach pain, vomiting, and a poor appetite for meat. He had been without a physician and without any treatment for over a year, ever since Dr. Barry E. O'Meara (1786–1836) was forced to return to England for having accused Napoléon's custodians of mistreating their prisoner.

Napoléon's friends and relatives were no fools. Why was a pompous and inexperienced medico appointed to replace O'Meara? One historian adduces sheer superstition as the cause of the misguided choice. In this version, Cardinal Fesch was impressed by the reports of a visionary woman, a profoundly pious German who passed for having seen the Holy Virgin. This woman came to Fesch and told him that the Mother of God had announced to her that the emperor was no longer at Saint Helena. Angelic legions had freed him from his captors and miraculously transported him elsewhere. Exactly where, was a mystery that the deity did not disclose, but the most important part of the message was that soon the world would again hear from him.[41]

Count Las Cases (1766–1842) came back to France after having followed Napoléon in his exile and recorded his conversations with the great leader during 18 months. He heard from the cardinal the fantastic story and could hardly believe his ears. Yet he was assured, in all earnestness, that what the English gazettes, letters, and other documents were saying was untrue; it was an effort to dissimulate the embarrassing fact that the emperor was no longer in the power of his captors. This was certain, for it was information that came "from a higher authority." The great Bonaparte could not be so easily ensnared: many a time his foes thought they had surrounded him, only to be confounded when, suddenly, as if by magic, he appeared behind them to rip them apart with his invincible fury. This time it would be no different.

Such being the case, reasoned the cardinal, what did it matter what kind of physician was sent to Saint Helena? For all one knew, an arrant quack would do, since the presumptive patient was no longer there! So, Antommarchi is surprised, upon reporting to the English authorities at Saint Helena, to find out that the prisoner is still there. He is careful in his approach to his exalted patient. He has heard that some of his predecessors got into trouble by insisting on diagnoses that were not acceptable to the English authorities. Dr. John Stokoe, for instance, arrived in June 1817 and had to depart in September 1819 largely because he diagnosed a hepatic problem in Napoléon, which he attributed to insalubrious living conditions. Brucellosis, sometimes with liver involvement, was very common in Saint Helena, as the goat milk consumed there came from goats imported from Malta, where the disease was endemic. But Napoléon had no right to fall ill. The world had to see that the disgraced leader of the French was treated magnanimously by the victorious British.

Antommarchi, however, is not too finicky when it comes to diagnostic labels. He heard it said in England that all that the fallen emperor (or as he calls him, "the general") really needs is a little exercise. And he comes with preconceived ideas that are not going to change *simply* because they do not fit the facts. Reality was never a sufficient motive to alter one's most cherished preconceptions. Napoléon, who formerly needed very little sleep, now passes his days in a semilethargic state. "He is exaggerating," thinks his Corsican physician, who winks to the English physicians, who wink back at him, as people aware of the fact that the patient is using his symptoms for some political motive, perhaps to be sent back to Europe.

He must be prompted to some physical activity, that is all. Does the general complain of an intense pain on the right scapular area and say that it feels as if a dagger were piercing through his back? Bah! Constipation. It will soon go away.

Yet Napoléon's health is really deteriorating: he is febrile, vomits blood, passes dark-colored stools indicative of upper gastrointestinal bleeding, and is racked with abdominal pain so intense that it makes him squirm and toss fitfully in bed. But his physician is not there during the worst paroxysms. Antommarchi is a dawdler, always waggish, always joking, nonchalant, going to town or strolling about, or else he is in town in hot pursuit of some pretty girl. When he comes to visit his patient, he is usually in a hurry. He does not stop for more than a few minutes. He appears in the imperial chamber in casual dress, disheveled, and addresses the French officers Henri-Gratien Bertrand and Count Charles-Tristan de Montholon, who were part of the emperor's general council and have followed him in his exile, by their names pure and simple, familiarly, omitting their titles or any formulas of respect.

When Napoléon felt death approaching, he called a priest and told him, "I was born a Catholic. I wish to fulfill all the duties that this faith imposes." In fact, he was never religious, and his approach to religious matters often smacked of cynicism. But this is a momentous occasion. The day of reckoning has come. Everyone senses the imminence of the great man's end.

At this very solemn moment, Antommarchi had the tactlessness of trying to make a joke. A wrathful emperor still found the energy to castigate him verbally: "Your inanities tire me, monsieur; I could well forgive your levity and your lack of good sense, but a lack of heart, never. Get out of here!" Then, alone with his faithful valet de chambre, he praised the discretion and judiciousness of the priest, and, concerning the physician, he added this comment: "As for that imbecile, it is hardly worth my while to occupy myself with him. Has anyone ever been worse cared for than I by him?"[42]

At length, the man before whom the whole of Europe trembled fell into a coma, never to wake up again. He died on the fifth of May, 1821, at five forty-five in the afternoon. He was 51 years old. The autopsy was performed the next day, on a billiard table of the residence where he was lodged, hastily improvised as autopsy table.

We have described Antommarchi's character in some detail, to show that the man who performed the autopsy was not above snatching and keeping any part of the body that might have suited his interests or ambitions. But this would have been difficult, because there were 16 or 17 persons watching the proceedings. Among those present were Bernard and Montholon; 6 English military physicians; Hudson Lowe, the governor of Saint Helena; 2 valets de chambre at the service of Napoléon; Abbot Paul Vignali, who had given the last rites to the dying emperor; and 3 local physicians officially appointed as observers.

In front of all these people, Antommarchi made an incision and exposed the organs, showing them to the witnesses as if he were giving a demonstration to students. A large ulcerated and indurated lesion occupied a large part of the stomach. This was probably an ulcerated cancer. By the light of present-day information, the old theories of conspiracy and arsenic poison, which form a huge conglomerate in the literature on Napoléon, may reasonably be discarded. The evidence definitely points to cancer of the stomach as cause of death.[43] Napoléon himself, suspecting his disease was centered on the stomach, had expressed his wish that after the autopsy, this organ be examined by experts and their conclusions forwarded to his son, the "King of Rome," known after the fall of the French empire as Duke of Reichstadt. In a romantic gesture, the fallen emperor also wished that his heart be taken to his estranged wife, Empress Marie-Louise.

Neither of these wishes was accomplished. The English authorities had opposed the embalming of the body and now prohibited the shipment of any organs. In this they showed themselves eminently prudent. The symbolic power of dead bodies, or even separate bodily parts, is none the weaker for their lifelessness. History shows that relics have enkindled the fervor of the masses, and corpses have mobilized hosts of men to dreadful feats of fanaticism and revolt. Of this there are vivid examples in our own times: to wit, the fierce clashes of political parties over the dead body of Evita Perón in Argentina or the daily televised images of Middle Eastern crowds inflamed to bloody revenge by the sight of the dead body of one of their comrades. Who knows what uncontrollable, furious stirrings might have been awakened, had Napoléon's heart, not to say his whole cadaver, come into the hands of his devoted followers. Thus, the desiccated stomach and heart were put into respective silver vases containing alcohol and placed by the body of the dead hero. They were there when the body was returned to France in 1840.

So much for the heart and the stomach displayed by Antommarchi. Other viscera ended up as part of a collection in the Museum of the Royal College of Surgeons of England. But what about the allegedly snatched penis? After Antommarchi had begun to sew the corpse with needle and string, everyone left the improvised autopsy room except the physician and the two faithful valets of the deceased emperor. One of them, Ali (Louis Etienne St. Denis), wrote in his memoirs that Dr. Antommarchi, before completing the suturing, "seizing the moment when the eyes of the English were not fixed upon the cadaver, extracted from a rib two little pieces [of tissue] that he gave to Monsieur Vignali and to Coursat [*sic*]."[44] The latter, Jacques Coursot (with an *o*) was the butler, and the former the abbot who administered the last rites to the dying Bonaparte. Vignali received, in gratitude for his many kindnesses to the fading emperor, several souvenirs, including plates, knives, forks, books, vases, a white shirt, and a handkerchief with the embroidered arms of Napoléon, in addition to his mortuary mask. Presumably, the "little piece of tissue," said to be taken from a rib, is what some have taken to be the dead man's phallus.

Historians have taken the trouble of tracing the fate of the objects bequeathed to Vignali. The abbot returned to his native Corsica. There he succumbed to one of those bloody vendettas for which his land was notorious: an old blood feud between families was the cause of his assassination in 1836. All his properties passed to his descendants, who, in 1916, sold the Napoleonic collection to an English booksellers' firm, Maggs & Co. An American physician, A. S. W. Rosenbach, of Philadelphia, bought it eight years later for $2,000. Among the various objects was the so-called mummified penis, which had been placed inside a leather box lined with blue velvet. The physician put it on display at the Museum of French Art in New York; visitors at the exhibit saw an object that "looked like

a maltreated buckskin shoelace or a shriveled eel."[45] Twenty years
later, the collection appeared in the hands of a Donald Hyde, and
upon his death it was sold to John Fleming. Next, in 1969, still
another collector, Bruce Gimelson, bought the Vignali bequeathal,
this time for the sum of $3,500. He tried to auction the objects
at Christie's of London, but he failed, there being no substantive
bids. (A British tabloid recounted the sale's failure with a humorous
headline in big, bold letters: "NOT TONIGHT, JOSEPHINE!")
However, eight years later, on October 26, 1977, a purchaser was
found at Drouot's auction house of Paris, who acquired several
items of the collection, now catalogued as lot 54 and described in
the following terms: "Tendon, head hairs and beard hairs [*cheveux
et poils de barbe*] taken from the body of the Emperor at the time of
his autopsy and given to Abbot Vignali. We attach a letter of abbot
Vignali, where he lists these tendon, head hairs, and beard hairs."[46]

The purchaser of lot 54 was John K. Lattimer, professor
emeritus of urology at Columbia University, who collected military objects, including some of a rather sinister hue, such as the
blood-stained collar that had belonged to President Lincoln, and
an ampoule of cyanide belonging to Nazi leader Hermann Göring.
Dr. Lattimer died on May 10, 2007, in Englewood, New Jersey.
As a professor of urology, he ought to have known what a penis
looks like. Yet considerable doubt exists over the true nature of
the Napoleonic tissue in his possession. A fragment of erectile
tissue pickled in liquid fixative for more than 100 years is not
likely to retain a fresh, easily identifiable appearance. French authors incline toward skepticism after having interrogated the officers who certified the authenticity of the objects sold at the 1977

Parisian auction. A commissioner-appraiser, who was personally acquainted with Dr. Lattimer, remembered that the tissue in lot 54 was a shriveled object, not much more than one inch in size, "and which could be nothing other than a fragment of rib," precisely as stated in the Vignali letter, which came also in the lot.[47]

Other published accounts are just as questionable. An American physician, Stanley M. Bierman, wrote an article in a medical journal describing the presumed posthumous vicissitudes of Napoléon's penis.[48] This author cites as the source of much of his information a popular book, *Auction Madness* by Charles Hamilton,[49] in which the extraordinary claim is made that Ali, Napoléon's manservant, had seen "unmentionable parts" of the body of the emperor being taken away by Abbot Vignali at the time of the autopsy. Both Bierman and Hamilton contend that Ali wrote down this observation and published it in an article in the prestigious literary French magazine *Revue de deux mondes* in 1852. However, no such article was seen after a careful perusal of all the issues of that publication for the mentioned year.

In sum, it appears that the identity of the controversial tissue is by no means ascertained. Dr. Lattimer's motives have been called into question. He declared his willingness to return the anatomical fragment to its rightful resting place—that is, next to the bodily remains of its owner, inside the coffin at the Invalides. He even suggested, in order for the French authorities to take his offer seriously, that the modern techniques of molecular biology be applied to the tissue fragment. Today DNA testing is profitably done on ancient biologic specimens, and the results are able to establish with a high degree of accuracy the paternity of a tissue sample. (Genomic testing would identify the tissue as belonging to

Napoléon, but microscopic examination of a biopsy might establish its origin from penis, and not from rib or chest wall.)

Some may see in all this nothing but a scheme concocted by Professor Lattimer to attract the attention of the public onto himself and his collection. Others would uncharitably label him a fetishist. Ultimately, whether the tissue he owned came from the copulatory organ of the emperor of the French, or not, is a supremely irrelevant question. Worthier of the attention of scholars is the obscure pulsation whence springs the desire to collect objects.

Collecting does not seem a trivial act (still more: ever since the 19th century, Freud accustomed us to think that there is no such thing as a trivial act). The Freudian exegesis pretends that behind our seemingly innocuous gestures and everyday activities lurk we know not what abysses of thwarted sexuality or libido gone awry. We may resist such interpretations, but when the collected object is a penis, with its heavy symbolic baggage of power, generation, fertility, virility, aggressiveness, domination, and life-giving energy, it is difficult not to think that those who would appropriate it are trying to arrogate to themselves the qualities they perceive as inherent in the collected object. Or perhaps they think it possible to vicariously compensate for their own sexual deficiencies by expropriating the severed sexual organs of famous men.

The Mad Monk's Mentula

In 2004 Igor Knyazkin, Russian sexologist and urologist and chief of the Prostate Center of the Russian Academy of Natural Sciences, proudly announced the opening of a museum of erotica in St. Petersburg, Russia. He had been collecting objects of erotic significance for decades, and had amassed more than 15,000 such

items; enough to be displayed, duly arrayed, in appropriate museum windows. Thus, he declared that Russia no longer had to envy
other countries in this regard: not Sweden, nor Denmark, known
for its liberal approach to sexual matters. Not Barcelona, Berlin,
or Prague, all of which boast respective exhibits of this kind. Not
even France, whose erotic museum occupies a seven-floor building
and opens to the public until two o'clock in the morning! No, sir.
Russia now had its own museum, its rich collection including the
penis of the famous court intriguer, Rasputin. And with a touch of
patriotic hauteur, he boasted that "Napoléon's organ is a mere 'pod'
in comparison with our thirty-centimeter-long organ."[50]

Grigori Efimovich Rasputin remains one of the most fascinating among the dark personalities of world history. The exact date of
his birth is unknown; it is given as 1869, 1870, or 1872. The place
was the village of Pokrovskoye in the remote Tyumen district of
Siberia. Here his conduct was soon infamous. Some have said that
Rasputin means "depraved," but this is because the word is similar
to the Russian *rasputny*, for "licentious" or the "debauched one." Be
that as it may, the man grew to act in perfect accordance with such
a designation. A tendency to mysticism is not incompatible with
outrageous libertinage, at least in certain temperaments. As an act
of penance for a theft or an act of vandalism, he made a pilgrim-
age to Verkhoturye Monastery. Presumably, he had a vision of the
Mother of God and was persuaded by a hermit at the monastery
to become a *strannik*, a religious pilgrim or a wanderer. As such, he
traveled through Greece and the Holy Land.

Rasputin never occupied a formal position in the organized
church, but the people learned to recognize him as a *starets*: an

elder or a man of wise counsel. He was almost illiterate but had a highly developed memory and an uncanny ability to quote Scripture in a most effective, dramatic way. He sympathized with the sect of the *Khlysty*, or flagellants. Again, there is no evidence that he ever joined that group, but it is easy to see why he liked them: rumor had it that they combined sexual experiences with their religious rituals.

On December 29, 1903, Rasputin became a student at the religious Academy of St. Petersburg, where he was introduced by his mentors to important people of the czar's court. One of these was the Grand Duchess Militsa, who happened to be one of the many devotees of esoteric and mystical religious sects then in fashion among the aristocracy. In turn, she introduced him to her sister Anastasia, and thus Rasputin gained direct access to court circles, where his demeanor as a tempestuous mystic, a rough-hewn *starets*, or an "illuminated," was bound to earn him a number of followers.

No small impression must have been caused by this outlandish, tall, wide-eyed, charismatic, semiliterate peasant and wandering mystic, who could utter apocalyptic, troubling speeches as if impelled by otherworldly fire. It so happened that the czar's young heir, Alexei, was afflicted with hemophilia. The imposing self-styled prophet was brought to the boy when he was having a painful bleeding episode, and to everyone's major astonishment, the crisis promptly subsided. A common version states that Rasputin used hypnosis. The physicians in attendance had been powerless to attenuate the young patient's suffering. It is highly improbable that bleeding may be stopped by hypnosis alone, but as everyone knows, the mind may work wonders upon the body. If not the bleeding, the severe distress, the pain, and the anxiety that accompanied the blood loss were dramatically arrested. Nothing more was needed for Czar Nicholas II and his czarina to feel profoundly indebted to the unkempt, moody mystic and to lavish upon him all sorts of rewards.

His ascent at court was not without obstacles. Pyotr Stolypin (1862–1911), the prime minister, ordered him out of St. Petersburg, much to the czarina's chagrin. However, Stolypin had his own problems, owing in large part to his ruthless suppression of peasants. He was assassinated coming out of the Kiev Opera Theater, a tragedy said to have been foretold by the wild-eyed mystic. Rasputin could then come back to exert a growing influence upon the ruling couple. By that power that a strong mind exerts upon the weak—a power as invariable as a natural law—the "mad monk," as Rasputin is sometimes called (an inaccurate nickname, since he was never a monk), came to acquire an inordinate control over the affairs of the state. He alone, among all members of the court, could bring relief to the young czarevich. In consequence, the mother, Czarina Alexandra, worshipped him as a healer, a holy man, "almost a Christ." The czar, no little influenced by his consort's opinion, saw in the figure of the long-haired, unkempt mystic a redemptor, "the voice of the downtrodden people."

Through Rasputin's influence, Russia did not enter the Balkan War of 1912–1913. All important posts in the government, not excluding the highest ministries, were owed to his good offices at court. Throngs curried his favor. Followers, admirers, and visitors came to his apartment at 64 Gorokhovaya Street, and it was no secret that his old concupiscent ways had only increased in proportion as his power and authority were augmented. In exchange for advancement at court, many of the distinguished ladies who solicited his attention balked not at yielding their charms to this uncouth seer, this mesmerizing prophet who addressed the highest aristocrat in an utterly familiar way, as if he were talking to a peasant. It was rumored that the czarina herself was among those fallen to the hypnotic powers of this uncommon man; evil tongues insinuated that she got from him more than spiritual guidance. In 1915, during the First World War, the czar organized his headquarters outside of St. Petersburg, placing his wife even more under the influence and psychological domination of Rasputin. This one could always count on the czarina to shield him from the effects of his profligacy and dissoluteness. For the ways of this crapulous, lecherous man were constantly the source of scandals.

All of this did not fall well with those who had reasons to resent his ascendancy. The czarina and Rasputin were accused by their enemies of being German agents during the war. A group of aristocrats headed by the young Felix Yusupov (1886–1967), who had married the czarina's niece, Princess Irina, conspired to assassinate the mad monk. Apparently, Irina, a woman of great beauty, was used as bait—unbeknownst to her—to bring Rasputin into the Yusupov palace.

His assassination is the stuff of legend. Under the pretext that Irina was going to arrive after some delay, Rasputin was ushered into a waiting room where the conspirators fed him cakes laced heavily with potassium cyanide. The volcanic soothsayer consumed some, yet showed no effect whatsoever. This alarmed and confused the would-be assassins. Yusupov then shot him with a revolver, and the other conspirators fell upon him and beat him mercilessly. But poison, blows, and gunshot wounds were apparently not enough to extinguish the life of this uncannily resilient giant. Yusupov's hand shook uncontrollably as he repeatedly fired on a victim that kept staring at him with fierce, flaming eyes—those eyes that so frightened the viewed. At length they wrapped his body, not yet completely exanimate, in heavy drapes and dropped him in the ice-filled river Neva. Only the cumulative action of poison, truncheons, bullets, and drowning brought forth the desired effect. Rasputin "finally" died on December 30, 1916.

Up to here, the narrated facts are generally accepted; from here on, the story loses verisimilitude. That the assassins may have mutilated the body in a murderous rage is appalling but not unbelievable. Historical examples abound in which castration was part of the punishment of a hated foe; during the French Revolution, irate mobs paraded the sex organs of dead aristocrats on the tip of swords or impaled on pikes—a cruel way chosen to signify that power and dominance had been violently snatched from the oppressors. But what then? In one implausible account, Rasputin's severed organ was left at the scene of the crime in the Yusupov palace, where a maid later found it "accidentally" while cleaning the room. Presumably, the maid handed over the "relic" to a group of the murdered mystic's admirers. These escaped to France during the Russian Revolution, and thus the admired phallus ended up in the possession of various collectors, whence it was recovered by the founder of the museum of erotica of St. Petersburg.

Much of this strains credibility. The documentary evidence is not nearly as profuse as that surrounding the death of Napoléon. Of course, it could not be, since the death of Rasputin was brought about by treacherous conspirators acting in stealth. To complicate matters, it has recently been contended that agents of the British Secret Service perpetrated the murder. A BBC *Timewatch* documentary aired on British television on October 1, 2004, claims that a reexamination of the original autopsy reports and Yusupov's version of the events revealed flagrant inconsistencies. This, together with memos uncovered in the files of the British Secret Service, maintains the documentary, is proof that the murder plot was commandeered and executed by the British, prompted by fears that Rasputin was about to pull Russia out of the war, thereby enabling the Germans to concentrate on the Western front and inflict major damage to Britain.[51]

The last word on the affair has not been told. Meantime, the mighty genital organ is displayed in the St. Petersburg museum. But just as the story is riddled with uncertainties, the actual specimen is clouded by doubts about its genuineness. It is a repulsive object that visitors to the museum can watch inside a jar of liquid fixative. The first reaction that its sight provokes is to ask how people can attain to such morbid vulgarity as to wish to see objects of this kind. The second, to wonder what sort of a hoax this is. For the dimensions of the thing displayed vastly exceed any recorded in the scientific literature. David Friedman's exhaustive review[52] included the neurotic exaggerations that fear of the black man's sexuality has inspired in white anthropologists. Even their prejudiced reports never described such penile hypertrophy: a long diameter of 11 inches, or nearly 30 centimeters in the flaccid state, is more than twice the highest figures on record. Not surprisingly, speculations about its true nature abound: some claim it is some wormlike marine being unfamiliar to most viewers, such as a sea cucumber (*Holothuroidea sp.*) or a geoduck (*Panopea abrupta*); others contend that it is the male organ of a horse or a bovine animal.

This activity may strike us as either revolting or fascinating. Yet public exhibition of the male sex organs of men who reach notoriety will continue. Such specimens will be coveted by collectors, and many of these will treat them like relics. In effect, the activities connected with these exhibitions are reminiscent of the medieval veneration of relics. And since the Middle Ages saw fit to confer the attributes of sainthood, including the capacity to work miracles, to each and every part of the body of saints, it is natural to ask whether the preternatural qualities were also extended to the sex organs. The answer is yes. I do not know of any place in the Catholic world where the erectile tissue of a holy man was ever worshiped in times past, but several traditions exist about the holy quality—nay, the godly nature—of a prepuce or foreskin. Striking as this may seem, the foreskin of Jesus Christ was once presented to the faithful as a holy relic.

The Prepuce of Jesus Christ

Jesus Christ was born a Jew; therefore he was circumcised at eight days of age, according to the ancestral custom. We read in Luke 2:21: "And when eight days were accomplished for the circumcising of the child, his name was called JESUS [. . .]" Surely, a part of the body of the Son of God could not be disposed of in an utterly casual manner. The prepuce, or foreskin, had to be most carefully preserved. During the Middle Ages, the monks of Coulombs, in the Diocese of Chartres, France, claimed to possess this holy relic. They exhibited what came to be known as "the holy prepuce," enchased in a silver reliquary. Its sight was welcomed specially by pregnant women,[53] in the belief that its beneficent action would make labor and delivery easier and painless. Apparently, King Henry V of England borrowed the sacred object in order to have his wife, Catherine of France, touch it, and then returned it to the monks.[54]

The priests of the Cathedral of Saint Etienne, in the Diocese of Châlons-sur-Marne, also claimed to have a part of the holy prepuce. Bishop Louis Antoine de Noailles (1651–1729), a powerful prelate who was made Peer of France, became head of the diocese in 1680. He was upset by what he considered a scandalous worship of the relic, above all by women, and decided to investigate the matter. He ordered the relic to be brought to him. It was wrapped in red velvet. A surgeon, as a person familiar with cut human tissues, was ordered to open the package, and all that was found inside was a little powder. Medicine at that time did not have at its disposal much in the way of analytical laboratory instrumentation; medical men relied mostly on their senses for diagnosis. Accordingly, the surgeon placed some of that powder under his tongue. After a moment's pause, he declared that it was nothing but ordinary house dust. This is how the so-called holy prepuce of Châlons-sur-Marne disintegrated into thin air.[55] Knowing that among today's Frenchmen a favorite fast-food snack is called the *croque-monsieur* (a grilled ham and cheese sandwich), we can appreciate the humor of their ancestors, who, starting from the described incident, applied to that surgeon the nickname of *croque-prepuce*.

Another holy prepuce was supposed to be in the basilica of Charroux, Diocese of Poitiers, in France. Presumably, it was brought there by an angel who gave it to the Byzantine Empress Irene of Athens, who gave it to Emperor Charlemagne in the late 8th century as a wedding gift. There were some who affirmed that the very name of Charroux came from an ancient locution that later evolved to *chair-rouge*, meaning "red flesh," to indicate that the holy relic, in spite of the time that had passed, preserved its reddish color—showing that it remained as fresh as at the time it was lopped off from the male organ of Our Savior. But erudite etymologists can always count on the existence of contrary factions. Thus it is that rival erudites, reading the ancient documents that deal with this subject matter, read *praesepium* (in Spanish, *pesebre*) instead of *preputium*—that is, "manger" instead of prepuce, and therefore their interpretation of the stories is entirely different. In that case, the relic kept there would be a piece of the holy manger, Christ's birthplace, not of the holy prepuce. The question is not solved, but the interest of the masses has waned, and nobody talks abut the holy prepuce of Charroux any more.

Whatever the case may be, how did the holy prepuce reach the Christian lands that revered it? I was quite fortunate in coming across the Spanish translation of a remarkable Italian book that picks up a tradition dating from the 13th century, where this matter is discussed. It is entitled *Evangelical Propinomio, or Evangelical Resolutions*, by an Augustinian prelate of the province of Lombardy, Donato Calvi of Bergamo.[56] The term *Propinomio* was apparently coined by the author, by combining the words *proper* and *name*, since the aim of the work was to establish the real identity of persons and things mentioned in Holy Scripture. Although the story dates from the 13th century, the Spanish book is from the first half of the 18th, and from the narrated facts, it is obvious that many additions and emendations were done to the text in the course of time. The subject of the holy prepuce is treated in a way that quaintly mixes fact with legend. The main points are developed as summarized next.

Calvi begins by telling us that in the ancient law, there were no ministers specifically appointed to perform circumcisions. Therefore, this task fell to oneself, or, in the case of children, to their fathers or mothers; there were no gender prohibitions. Thus, Abraham circumcised himself, and Sephora, the wife of Moses in the book of Exodus, circumcised their second son, Eliezer. Calvi then quotes Saint Hilarion's version that Christ was taken to the Jerusalem temple to be circumcised, but promptly rules out this hypothesis because, according to the ancient Mosaic law, infants could not be taken to the temple before reaching the age of 40 days. We are then told that the most plausible explanation is found in a text from Saint Epiphanius of Salamis in his book *Adversus Haereses* (*Against Heresies*), which says that Christ was circumcised in the very same spot where he was born, namely in a manger of Bethlehem (*Christus natus est in Bethlehem, circumcisus in spelunca . . .*). Authority is also appealed to, since we are told that the Fathers of the Church all sanction this version.

It remains only to determine whether it was the patriarch Saint Joseph or the Holy Virgin Mary who performed the surgical excision. Our author first quotes the writings of Saint Jerome favoring the former, then those of Saint Bernard inclining to the latter. This second opinion he deems most probable because it used to be customary to delegate this task to the mothers, who, on account of the love and tenderness they felt for their children, would tend to "use the knife with greatest care and inflict upon them the least pain." But also, he says, since "Mary had given flesh and blood to the Son without any admixture of male, it was most fitting that she should be the first to spill that blood for the sake of the salvation of humankind."

What happened next? Mary, says our chronicler, kept that "beloved treasure with her until her happy transit" out of earthly life. Then, in one version, she bequeathed it to Saint John the Evangelist, and in another to Saint Mary Magdalen. Angels—who else?—then transported the sacrosanct relic to Emperor Charlemagne, who ordered it placed in a temple in Poitiers (Charroux, apparently). In Calvi's version, however, the relic did not stay there but was transported to Rome, the center of the Catholic faith, for it to repose in the Lateran Basilica, where it was duly kept for many years.

But repose is not appointed for things that dwell among human beings. The sacrosanct foreskin was undisturbed until the year 1527. On May 6 of that year, the troops of Emperor Charles V, having defeated the French army and its allies in Italy, who supported the anti-Spanish Pope Clement VII against the emperor, sacked Rome. Upset for lack of pay, the wild soldiery ran over Rome pillaging, killing, destroying art works, torturing men, and raping women. The palaces of high prelates of the church were set to ruin, their treasures vandalized or stolen. Even those cardinals and bishops who had favored the emperor had to run for their lives. The Lateran Basilica was not exempt from the depredations. A soldier stole the holy prepuce together with other relics.

This soldier had fled into the village of Calcata—a place under the feudal power of the Anguillara family, about 20 miles from
Rome—when he was arrested by the local authorities and imprisoned. Afraid of being punished for a crime against religion, not just
for a simple theft (at the time, the cruelest tortures were inflicted
upon the sacrilegious), he managed to hide the relic in the basement of the castle, where he was locked. At length he was freed,
and, finding himself on the point of dying, he confessed his theft
to the priest who was giving him the last rites. This one relayed
the story to Pope Clement VII, who in turn wrote to Giovanni
Battista Anguillara, Lord of Calcata, Stabbia, and Massano, advis-
ing him to search for the sacred relic. But the indications given by
the soldier had been imprecise; the search was fruitless.

Thirty years later, in 1557, it pleased heaven to satisfy the pious
desires of the faithful. A visiting priest entered the basement where
the relic was hidden. Although looking for something else, he fortuitously discovered the precious object. It was inside a steel box
"long of about half a palm and tall of about four fingerbreadths."
He took it to a respected lady, Magdalena Strozzi, who at the time
resided in Stabbia. The lady opened the box in the presence of the
priest as well as Lucretia Orfini (wife of the lord of the castle) and
her eight-year-old daughter, Chiara. They found inside three relics
wrapped in parchment with inscriptions that were almost illeg-
ible, so worn out were they. One was a piece of the flesh of Saint
Valentine Martyr "the size of a walnut, and so fresh that it seemed
recently cut." The second was a fragment of the mandible, with a
tooth, of Saint Martha, sister of Saint Mary Magdalen. The third
was inscribed "Jesus." Lady Magdalena Strozzi attempted to undo

the knot in the thread that tied the wrapping but could not do it. Her hands seemed as if paralyzed; she could not move them, and the rest of the persons present looked on silently in amazement and fright.

Magdalena Strozzi loudly implored heaven with prayers and acts of contrition to allow her to open the sacred bundle. All to no avail. Then, as those present started to break down in sobs and tears, the lady Orfini exclaimed, "This must certainly be the container that holds the prepuce of Our Redeemer, for I remember that Pope Clement VII wrote a letter to Giovanni Battista, my husband, precisely about this matter!" No sooner had she pronounced these words than an exquisite fragrance was diffused throughout the room and invaded the whole castle.

Perplexed by all these marvels, they did not know what to do, until the good priest suggested to let the little girl, Chiara, open the bundle, since her innocent hands might be permitted to perform the required maneuver. They agreed, and immediately after the girl touched the string, the knot became miraculously undone, the package opened, and the holy prepuce was exposed. "It was curled, dense, and of the color and size of a chickpea," says Calvi. They put it inside a new small bag, replaced it in the steel box with the other relics, and transported it to the church of Calcata, where it was deposited on the altar to saints Cornelius and Cyprian.

A great number of miracles were attributed to the presence of the holy relic. The nuns of St. Ursula, from the neighboring hamlet of Massano, were warned by divine inspiration of the arrival of the holy prepuce and came walking and carrying lighted torches to visit the church of Calcata, where it was kept. The relic was

mysteriously enveloped by a mist seeded with dazzling, scintillat-
ing stars. The crowds desirous to see the relic were so dense that
many people climbed on the roof of the church and removed the
tiles in order to be able to contemplate the sacred object (or, I am
to assume, at least the box in which it was kept).

There is no point in recounting the many portents that are
consigned in hagiography and legend in connection to this relic.
I will finish this narrative by adding that the general commotion
originated by the presence of the holy object in Calcata reached the
ears of the reigning Pope Paul IV (ruler from 1555 to 1559), who
sent two clergymen to find out the circumstances of the matter
and to decide on the authenticity or spuriousness of the relic. The
two canons, Cenci and Pipinelli, conducted the appropriate investigations and concluded in favor of the legitimacy of the find; their
official report, signed on May 1, 1559, said that without a doubt,
the real prepuce of Our Lord was at Calcata. Except that in the
course of carrying out their investigations, Pipinelli had wished to
test the elasticity of the object, and no better way of doing this occurred to him than to stretch it by hand. (Again, the rudimentary
technology of the times precluded any more sophisticated testing.)
He did this so strongly that, alas, the prepuce tore into two fragments. Immediately the air grew foggy, darkness descended upon
the earth, and lighting shot out of the sky so loud and so threatening "that it seemed Judgment Day had arrived."

At one time, about a dozen medieval European sanctuaries
claimed to have a fragment of the holy prepuce: Lorraine, Metz,
Châlons-sur-Marne, Charroux, Antwerp, Santiago de Compostela,
Hildesheim, Coulombs, and Le Puy-en-Velay, among of the.

One could propose a miraculous elasticity of the sacred foreskin allowing all these sites to possess a fragment of the relic, but this hypothesis is untenable, as clearly shown by the unfortunate Pipinelli accident. The fact is, the church recognized the unbecoming nature of this cult and, by a decree of 1900, strictly prohibited to speak of this relic or to foster its cult and veneration in any way. The holy prepuce may still be in Calcata, but it will not be taken out from seclusion and never again will it be shown to visitors.

It is not difficult to see in medieval legends and stories a certain charm and freshness that our jaded times painfully lack. Even when, as in the cult of relics, fanaticism incurred undesirable excesses, it is still possible to detect a certain underlying pulsation of vitality and human warmth that one would look for in vain in today's social manifestations. Six or seven centuries ago, the contours of life stood more marked than today. As the medievalist Johan Huizinga put it in his well-known book, *The Waning of the Middle Ages*, pleasure and pain were felt more violently then; every experience, every event, and every action had the "directness and absoluteness" that pleasure and pain still have for the mind of a child.[57] Our epoch came up with a contemporary equivalent of relic worship that could not be more drab and uninspired: I mean the commercialization of human parts that are sold at auctions.

Penile tissues will continue to be treated in this way, however vulgar or displeasing it may seem, for the symbolism of this anatomical part remains very strong. The penis lives forever in the collective imagination as a blind force, a creative principle, the power of vegetative life, the conduit of virile might. In our unconscious, does it not seem inevitable to attribute a magic nature to an object that transmutes from a silky, softish, quiescent presence into a rigid, aggressive, willful huntsman's tool? And to our conscious awareness, it represents the source of man's physical pleasure, but also—a fact most evident to those familiar with human pathology—the cause of physical and spiritual pain and unbearable anguish. Artists have known the ambivalence of the male sex organ by intuition. Michel Tournier, a contemporary French writer, spoke of it in his novel *Les Météores* as "a paradoxical fountain," for it discharges alternatively urine and semen—that is, now the ammoniacal liquid that is like a distillate of all the body's impurities, the effluent that removes toxic products, now the fluid that is the vehicle for life's creation, the very sap that sustains the existence of the human race.

I cannot avoid being moved by this paradox: a "fountain" from which flows at times—but only sporadically—the quintessence of all that is delectable, luxuriant, prolific, and orgiastic; and at other times—regularly, several times a day—the fluid that carries the waste that results from the process of our daily dissolution: the mark of our gradual wreckage and progressive, irrevocable march toward death.

Cardiovascular

Which Comes First, the Head or the Heart?

The heart, as everyone knows, is a muscular organ situated in the thorax, between the two lungs. The question is, how did this organ come to represent in the collective imagination—throughout the whole world—the seat of passions, of sensibility, and generally of affect and emotions? For, in all the languages, the heart is assigned a sort of metaphorical destiny that is invariably magnanimous or grandiose. Goodness and altruistic sentiments such as charity, compassion, devotion, and pity are made to reside in the heart, since we say that a person endowed with these virtues has "a big heart" ("a heart as big as all outdoors," says an American hyperbolic phrase) or is "good hearted." We receive "with all our heart" that for which we feel a warm sympathy. We "set our heart upon" what we earnestly desire, but if our wish is thwarted, disappointment "breaks our heart," or we brood silently, "eating our heart out."

But not only affection and emotions reside in the heart. Cognition, perception, and understanding are faculties over which the heart has long vied with the brain. Thus, we say we "learn by heart" that which we commit to memory or have understood thoroughly. And note, further, that the heart is believed to make possible a higher form of cognition, a level of understanding superior to that acquired by the brain. "The heart has its reasons that reason itself does not know at all; we know this by a thousand ways," reads Pascal's famous pronouncement, meaning that the heart has access to a superior form of awareness barred to the intellect, for, as he pointed out, "It is the heart who feels God, not reason. There you have what faith is: God sensed by the heart, not by reason."[1]

I confess to a certain partiality for the "cognition of the heart," understood as knowledge strongly impregnated with emotion. An example from my own lived experience makes this point quite well. A journalist once asked me what I had learned, speaking not from a technical or medical point of view but as a human being, after a whole professional life spent as a pathologist. He wished to know what humanistic lesson, what "wisdom" had I derived from my many years of close contact with cadaver dissections. I felt utterly nonplussed. It was as if he had asked me, "Please resume for me, in the next ten seconds, what you think is the meaning and purpose of your existence."

I quickly ran through my mind the images of many human beings whose acquaintance I had made after they became corpses, and I could not avoid the melancholy reflection that their deaths had obeyed to inconsiderable, often trivial causes: the angelic four-year-old girl who collapsed in the physician's office after a penicillin injection and could not be resuscitated; the vigorous rancher who died from a pulmonary embolus after a minor hernia operation; the college student who succumbed from asphyxia due to a cocktail's olive lodged in his throat; the brawny, adventuresome fellow who survived a thousand dangerous exploits only to be felled by a tiny parasite tunneling through his vital organs. Then, in my perplexity, the first thing that came to my mind, by way of reply to the journalist's question, was: "What that experience taught me is how tenuous and transient are our lives." To which the man, undaunted, rejoined, "In that case, doctor, you learned nothing, since *that* we knew already."

This time my confusion was complete. I did not know what to say. Only later, after much thinking, I realized that my questioner had failed to make a crucial distinction. I mean discrimination between two forms of knowing: the two kinds of cognition often called, in metaphorical terms, understanding from the head and from the heart. From the head—that is, intellectually—we all know very well that life is fleeting and vulnerable. But this knowledge is a feeble and inchoate, and therefore inferior, form of knowledge. Only truly shaking experiences, such as seeing for the first time a human cadaver being dissected, or suffering bereavement, can deliver to us the full knowledge—the knowledge from the heart—about life's transitoriness and evanescence.

A purely intellectual cognition is a cool light. It bathes the objects of contemplation in its unambiguous limpidity but keeps us at a distance from them, as when we see museum specimens neatly arranged behind their display windows, which we soon forget. This kind of knowledge rarely moves us to action. Knowledge from the heart engages us, draws us to the world, and sears its stamp indelibly in our lives. For only when we get to know things viscerally, so to speak, can we say that we have learned them fully. As for me, the dead gave me the *knowledge from the heart*; the enhanced apprehension of this awful reality.

The head, of course, has been thought to have the chief place in determining our reactions. Throughout history, it was seen as the seat of a directive force. In most cultures, the brain was deemed to determine all our actions and, therefore, to configure the very core of individual personality. Scholars have proposed that the sinister practice of decapitation originated in the desire to destroy what is most intimate and fundamental in the person of the enemy, or else in the desire to forcibly remove and appropriate the foe's most valuable attributes, which some have located in the head: grit, courage, strength.

With the advent of Christianity, the symbolism of the head was lifted to very high levels. Christ was made into the head of the Church, while the latter was his body. Wrote Saint Paul in his letter to the Colossians, inhabitants of the ancient city of Colossae, in Phrygia (New Testament, Colossians 1:18): "He is the head of the body, the Church, the beginning, the first born from the dead, that in everything he might be preeminent." And Christ becomes (in Colossians 2:19) "—the Head, from whom the whole body, nourished and knit together through its joints and ligaments, grows with a growth that is from God."

Yet the heart never ceased to exert its unique fascination. It all started with Aristotle, who in his book *Generation of Animals*[2] affirmed that the heart is the first organ to be formed in the embryo (735a 20). When something grows, he reasoned, there must be something that makes it increase its growth. Hence, that which comes into being first must be able to increase the embryo, and from this it follows that the heart is "the first principle of a natural body" (738b 15). It is not true that the heart is the very first organ to be formed: a rudimentary alimentary canal is already present, but the Stagirite did not have the benefit of microscopy while examining embryos, and it is always striking to see with the naked eye, in chick embryos—a favorite model of all the early embryologists—the beating heart appear when other structures are barely discernible.

The ambiguities in medieval thought concerning the heart and the head are apparent in the work of the greatest encyclopedist of the Middle Ages, Saint Isidore of Seville (CA. 560–636). In his monumental opus, *Etymologies*,[3] he states: "The first part of the body is the head [*caput*], which received this name because all the senses and the nerves originate therefrom [*initium capiunt*], and all source of strength issues from it" (Book XI, 25). And of the heart he states: "The heart [*cor*] comes from a Greek voice named *kardian*, or of *cura* [care, concern]. In it resides all anxious thought and the cause of science [. . .] From it, two arteries come out. The left one has more blood, the right one more air [*spiritus*]. This is why we observe the pulse on the right arm" (Book XI, 118).

Thus, for Isidore, the heart, not the head, is the seat of knowledge, "the cause of science." It is true that all the evidence he adduces (preposterous to us, but dear to the scholastic intellectuals in the Middle Ages) is only his personal opinion about the origin of the words that denote the bodily organs. But he is clear about physiology, as understood in his time: "By the spleen we laugh, by the bile we are angry, by the heart we are wise, by the liver we love. And while these four elements remain [constant], the animal is whole." ("*Nam splene ridemus, felle irascimur, corde sapimus, iecore amamus. Quibus quattuor elementis constantibus integrum est animal*".) (Book XI, 127). It is interesting that the source of knowledge is, in Isidore's scheme, within the heart, whereas the seat of amorous sentiment he locates, of all places, in the liver.

Many ponderous volumes would be needed to describe the conflict between the head and the heart. By this I mean the clash of two philosophical attitudes: that which attributes predominance to thought and understanding, and that which affirms the primacy of emotion in our lives. The debate is perhaps idle by the light of modern psychology. Yet somehow it still seems pertinent to ask, at a very fundamental level, which comes first, the head or the heart; in other words, cognition or emotion.

Philosophers have framed this question in a provocative way: when in the course of our lives we encounter a new object, do we know it first, or do we like it first? This question may strike one as irrelevant, for how could we possibly like or dislike anything without knowing it first? That would be like putting the cart before the horse. But a little reflection may show that the question is not entirely senseless.

When we first look at an indifferent object, our eyesight glides over its surface, *apparently* in a random way. Take a blank page in a notebook. Our glance may stop, if only for an instant, at a corner of the paper, at a fold, or at the central fissure where two bound pages come together. On a building's bare wall, our eyes may first spot a little crack here or a slightly shaded area there. Leonardo da Vinci, like all the great painters, remarked that every object, even the most trivial and "uninteresting," possesses innumerable details that the human eye could not possibly apprehend simultaneously. (Furthermore, these details are always changing with movements and the displacement of the light source.) Yet it is a fact that our eyes stop preferentially here or there. This "preference" may be said to be gratuitous, since we don't "know" the object yet, but it is not random. It is rather a liking or a relishing; an inclination or partiality that is not the effect of reasoning, but depends entirely on our affect.

Stated differently, our eyes stop here or there simply because we "like" those details that catch our vision; this is purely a matter of the heart, before any conscious, rational evaluation of the object seen. Using the term in a broad sense, we may say that it is a matter of love. Immediately after the first fleeting impression, thought comes in, we judge the object before our eyes, and we may decide that we dislike it. But during the initial instant, however transient it may have been, our vision is guided purely by emotion devoid of intellection or rational activity. Metaphorically speaking, the heart comes first, the head second. In the order of things human, love is always primary: this is what Max Scheler (1874–1928) called the *ordo amoris*, love's order. This German philosopher contended that a whole realm of inner life, the great transcendence of which must not be disregarded, is related to facts that have nothing to do with thought and understanding. He who disregards this realm just because it is independent of thought "is like a man who has healthy eyes and closes them and wants to perceive colors with his ear or his nose."[4]

The Heart and Devouring Passion

Saint Augustine, one of the chief defenders of the primacy of the heart, made this organ the repository of spirituality. He felt that the noblest feelings and aspirations resided here. But by the 12th century, with the appearance of "courtly love," the heart became the domain of love, sacred as well as profane. It is not entirely clear why this was so, but as stated before, the ideas of the ancients—and particularly the biology and psychology propounded by Aristotle—had much to do with making the heart the seat of love. Arab translations of the Stagirite's works diffused these ideas throughout much of the known world during the Middle Ages. The textbooks of medicine, carefully preserved and edited by Arab physicians, described the amorous passion as a disease that affected chiefly the heart, although the original stimulation for this passion depended on the imaginative and perceptive faculties that resided in the brain.

No less influential in this regard were the works of the Fathers of the Church, whose reliance upon the metaphoric images of the heart as the seat of *caritas* (charity, particularly viewed as a Christian virtue) and divine love further reinforced the idea of the heart as the habitat of affect. To these factors must be added perhaps less momentous, but not insignificant, circumstances. For instance, it has been suggested that, in the language of the troubadours of the "courts of love," the words for heart and love—respectively *cor* and *amor*—have a similar sound that facilitated versification but at the same time contributed to establish the notion of the heart as the natural realm of love.

Once the idea was consolidated that love resides in the heart, the medieval aesthetic sensibility conceived a striking story that has survived across geographical borders and successive eras, down to the present time.[5] It is a story of passion, adultery, violence, and horrid vengeance. Its earliest European form is that of the "lay" (short lyrical poem) of Ignaure (*lai d'Ignaure*). It is attributed to a little-known composer, Renaut de Beaujeu, and dates from the late 12th or early 13th century. Its startling plot is described next.

Ignaure is a dashing knight, fond of jousting, and merrymaking, and, to his misfortune, quite a ladies' man. He finds himself in the castle of Riol, in Brittany, where 12 couples happen to be lodging at the time. The knights are 12 valorous men, each of whom has a lovely wife of the highest nobility and most graceful deportment. Ignaure loses no time and courts all the women, one after the other, each time promising fealty and devotion, and each time forgetting what he said to the one as soon as he approaches the other. Because he is a likeable fellow and much admired, his wooing prospers, and the ladies grant him their favors—each one showing herself tender and loving, persuaded that he belongs to her alone.

Then comes the day of Saint John, and a feast of merriment and general revelry. The ladies withdraw to a corner of the garden to play games. One of them suggests a game in which she would act the part of a priest, and all the rest would come to confession. They would confess the name of the man they love, to whom they have surrendered, and thus would find out who has the noblest and worthiest lover.

The ladies accept, and each one confesses to the "priest" that her lover is the most famous and valorous man, the flower of knighthood, Ignaure. Each time this name is pronounced, the listener pales. But, one after another, all the confessants utter the same name. When the last confession takes place, the fake priest smiles in spite of herself: the rascal whom she believed her devoted lover has been named 11 times; not one of the ladies gave a different name.

After the round of confessions is over, the women gather, curious to know who among them will be acknowledged as having the noblest, most desirable lover. They are shocked and irate to learn the truth from the lips of the game leader:

> "Ignaure is a traitor who has shamed us all. A curse upon him! I love him, too, just like all the rest of you. But he will pay dearly for what he has done to us."

> "How can we avenge ourselves?" asked her listeners.

> "I'll tell you how. The next one to hear his advances will give him a rendezvous in this garden. Then she will notify us all, and we shall all be hiding at the time and place of the intended tryst. And make sure, each one of you, to bring with you a pointed steel knife with well sharpened edges. He is going to pay for the pain that he has caused us."

Unaware of the women's conspiracy, Ignaure is soon flattering and cajoling the belle that chances to be closest to him, as was his wont. The woman pretends to receive his sweet talk favorably, does not reject his embraces, and kisses him tenderly. But when his desire has been kindled, she stops him:

"Come see me at the corner of the garden that you know, next Sunday evening. There you will obtain the complete satisfaction of your desires."

Our man eagerly attends the assignation and is overjoyed to find the lady ever well disposed toward his advances, when, in the midst of the most sensuous caresses, he is suddenly startled to see the women appear from all sides, their faces red with anger and resentment.

"Is this a trap, my lady? Has an ambush been prepared?"

The women surround him, threateningly, all with knives hidden under their mantles, but the knight finds the resolve to tell them:

"Be welcome, ladies, all of you."

"To your undoing," they answer. "For you shall not leave this place until you have received the recompense that is due to a traitorous, false, and disloyal villain."

The woman who had played the part of a priest speaks then:

"Allow me to be the first to speak, and afterwards each one will say whatever she wants. Ignaure, do not lie to me at this moment. For a long time, I had been your friend, and I had surrendered my heart to you."

"My lady, I am always your friend, your vassal, and your servant knight. And yours is my heart, loyally and wholly."

Upon hearing this reply, one of the women advances full of spite and anger, and says:

"You wretch! You knave! Were you perchance not *my* lover?"

"Yes, my lady, that I was. And God is my witness that I will always be, since my heart never failed you, and my love for you will never weaken."

Another woman looks at him full of jealousy and says:

"Woe is me! Damned betrayer! Those are the very words you did address to me. And you now love another woman, not me? This, after having sworn that you would always be mine?"

"My lady, I love you truly, and my love for you shall be ever faultless."

Upon which, still another woman exclaims:

"What! Had you not promised to love *me* without fault?"

"Yes, my lady. I did promise, and I do love you, and I love all of you with all my strength, just as I love your games and your pleasures."

Writes the author of the narrative: "You should have heard what a ruckus, what a din was then caused by the women! And what screams, what irate disputes and what threats converged upon the noble knight!" The women's knives then came out, together with this terrible menace:

"Ignaure, your conduct toward us has been so evil, that you are going to die this very minute. God alone could save you."

Undaunted, our man replies:

"Ladies, be not so cruel, and please abstain from committing so great a sin. Were I to find myself now with my helmet tied in place, astride on a war steed, a shield guarding my left arm, and my sword firmly held in my right hand, I would dismount right here and surrender myself to your mercy. For I am sure that if I were to be slain by such beautiful hands, I would become a martyr and would dwell amidst the saints in paradise; I know I was born under a lucky star."

The feminine heart is tender. We are to suppose that words of this kind found their way into the hearts of the listeners, with the effect of softening their murderous resolve and turning it to tears. There follows a deliberation among them, and, if not the full forgiveness of their grievances, at least the suppression of their murderous intent. Then the lady who had played the part of priest addresses the wily knight:

"Ignaure, you deceived us well until we discovered your slyness. We can no longer love you in the same way as before. But we have decided to let you choose. The woman you prefer will keep you, for each woman wishes to have a lover who would be hers only."

"By no means! I mean to continue loving all of you, as I have done heretofore."

"Do as I order you, Ignaure, or I swear, by my head, that you shall not come out of here alive. Take the one you want."

This is strong persuasion. The knight feels compelled to answer: "My lady, I choose you. I am unhappy to renounce the love of all the other ladies, for they all have great qualities, but it is your love that attracts me the most." And upon this reply, the women, although frustrated and saddened, swear amongst them that they would leave him and his chosen lady alone, and go back to their homes.

(Such generosity in a cohort of spited and jealous women? Unbelievable, but we are not about to quibble with a poet).

Things might have settled in this newly obtained placidity, but perhaps it was foreordained that it should not be so. A meddlesome man, as crafty as he was knavish, had been present in the garden and overhead all the proceedings. With his characteristic, malicious shrewdness, he piques the curiosity of the knights residing in the castle by insinuating that he was the possessor of a secret that concerned them all. They implore him to disclose it in exchange for some money. He first exacts from them the oath that they would not harm him, and, feeling secure, he tells them the entire story.

"The man has made cuckolds of the whole lot of you. But now he is master of the wife of only one man."

"Which one? Do you know him?"

And the informer, addressing one man in particular, says, "It is you." To which the man replies, "By God! Why, if I am the husband, I am luckier than the rest."

The men swear that no one would say a word of what had transpired there; they warn the spy that his life would be in danger if he spoke of this to anyone else, pay him his money, and dismiss him. They stay in the room, trembling with ire, to plan their vengeance.

The husband of the lady who had played the part of the priest promises that he would have spies watch every movement of the lovebirds, so as to surprise them in the act. This was not difficult. Now that Ignaure has been reduced to illicit monogamy, he pays his visits to a single lady. The chronicler quaintly writes: "The mouse that lives in only one hole will sooner fall into the trap!" Indeed, the aggrieved husband is soon informed that the knight and his wife were together. He knew that an underground passage of the castle communicated with his wife's bedroom, took this passageway, and emerged fully armed, catching the two lovers in bed. The adulterous knight realizes that he was doomed. All he can say is:

> "Sir, have pity on us! You can see that we truly love each other. I have committed a great fault against you, and I know there is no way to excuse it or hide it."

The lady is desperate and implores her husband to spare Ignaure. Her pleading is to no avail. The outraged husband takes the knight away and locks him up in a dungeon, under the constant watch of trustworthy jailers. Meanwhile, the lady expresses an immense pain, looks pale, cries, sobs, and pulls her hair until whole tufts come out in her hands. When she regains some composure, she informs the rest of the women of what had happened. She asks for their solidarity: "Just as we shared him in pleasure, so our pain must now be common to all!"

Their natural tenderness and sympathy wins again the upper hand. They wished to know what had happened to Ignaure, and upon meeting with the silence of their spouses, they declare that they would touch no food until they would find out whether Ignaure was dead or alive. From then on they fast.

The offended husband who had captured Ignaure calls his companions and proposes to them a manner of vengeance. He tells them:

"All these contemptible, depraved women have promised to fast until they know whether the man will die or will be spared. Four days hence, we shall kill him, cut his male member, the bodily part that gave them so much pleasure, and his heart too, for good measure; and with these organs we shall prepare a food that we shall, by using trickery, make them eat. I can think of no better vengeance!"

This heinous crime is carried out as planned. The men kill the knight, castrate him, extract his heart, and prepare a savory dish with these organs. Then they announce to their wives that he is alive and has been freed. Next they present to them the carefully prepared food and use all manner of blandishments and flattery to make them eat. The ladies, who had fasted several days, are especially sensitive to their entreaties. They eat to satiety.

The husband who had surprised the lovers in flagrante delicto asks his wife if she liked the dish. She naively answered that she could hardly remember anything more delicious and satisfying. Her husband rejoins:

"My lady, you have eaten what you were so avid for, those things that made your contentment so fully, that you desired nothing else. I have killed your lover and cut him to bits; and you and all your women friends have partaken of the very things for which you used to be gourmands. Did you have enough, all twelve of you? Now our affront has been avenged."

When the disloyal wife hears this terrifying account, she loses consciousness. As soon as she recovers her senses, she sends messengers to the other women, to inform them of what had happened. They decide they would never eat again, and pass their time in lamentations, evoking the image of their disappeared paramour, wringing their hands, and crying most piteously. "The pain they demonstrated," says the chronicler, "was such that those who heard them cried too. They became weaker and weaker for lack of food, but heeded not the implorations of friends and relatives who exhorted them to eat. The death of the twelve ladies was mourned, and a lay in twelve verses was composed, which must be remembered, because the story is true."

This grim, sanguinary narrative must have touched a raw nerve of the European sensibility, because the story has been repeated across countries and down the ages under various guises. It is intriguing that the women should have been 12, like the Apostles. The fact that they share the flesh of their lover is not without troubling Eucharistic reminiscences. The lay of Ignaure's sources are obscure. Some scholars have hypothesized that its theme is of Celtic origin, given the known partiality of Celtic bards for stories of guilty love and ferocious vengeance. On the other hand, there are ancient Oriental narratives in which the heart is represented as the seat of passions, emotions, and sexual desire. These include an Egyptian legend in which a young man, fleeing the turpitude that would turn him into the culpable lover of his own brother's wife, castrates himself and takes out his own heart.[6] This story goes back to the remotest antiquity, antedating even the Greek myth of the dismembering of the god Dionysus. It is among the oldest testimonies to the fact that widely separate world cultures have regarded the heart as the seat of passions, the principle of life, and the vital pulsation of sexuality.

Similarly, in an Indian story, the Rajah Rasalu of Punjab is out hunting in the woods, when his parrot flies to alert him about his wife's adultery. He comes back, kills the adulterous man, takes out his heart, and cooks with it a tasty fricassee that he and his wife eat with relish. (Narratives of this type often spare no details about the garnishing, sauces, condiments, side dishes, and other culinary refinements that compose the macabre menu.) When the rajah reveals to his wife the ingredients of the dish she has just eaten, she spits out the piece of meat that is still in her mouth but defiantly reproaches him for his cruelty, then hurls herself to her death from a high tower.[7]

Whether the story of the eaten heart traces its roots to the Orient or is indigenous to the West, certain it is that it became part of the cultural heritage of many Western nations. The Provençal legend of Guilhem de Cabestany (CA. 1240) reproduces the chief facts of Ignaure's lay: the husband murders his wife's lover and feeds her the slain man's heart, appropriately well condimented. She kills herself upon learning the horrific truth. Giovanni Boccaccio (1313–1375) retells the story in his famous *Decameron* (1351), where it appears as the tenth story of the fourth day, devoted to ill-starred lovers. Its long title summarizes the plot well:

"Sir Guglielmo Di Roussillon gives his wife to eat the heart of Sir Guglielmo Di Guardastagno, by him slain and loved of her, which she after coming to know, casts herself from a high casement to the ground and dying, is buried with her lover."

Each time the story is retold, variations are introduced in accordance with the author's character and aesthetic sensibility, the temper of the times, and the idiosyncrasies and conventions of the society to which the storyteller belongs. Dante, in his *La Vita Nuova* (III), dreams that his beloved eats his heart, although this does not happen in a context of jealousy and vengeance but is symbolic of the spiritual ravishment he experiences. In Germany, the legend of the minnesinger Reinmar von Brennenberg, at the closing of the 15th century, has the lover slain by the jealous husband, who then extracts his heart and feeds it to his wife, even though the illicit love had never reached consummation. The female author, Madame d'Aulnoy (née Marie-Catherine Le Jumel de Barneville, 1650–1705) places the story in a Spanish setting and makes a woman, the wife of the Marquis of Astorga, assassinate her husband's mistress. In this case, it is the faithless husband who unwittingly consumes the heart of his lover in a ragout. Nor is this appalling viciousness enough. The wife, having gone mad from jealousy, throws the bloodied head of her victim, which she was hiding under her ample skirt, on top of the table where her husband dined with some friends. She ends her days locked up in a convent, while her husband sinks into a profound depression.[8]

Scholars have traced the persistence of the legend of the eaten heart from antiquity through the Middle Ages, the Renaissance, the Baroque period, the Enlightenment, Romanticism, and the 20th century, down to the present time.[9] This remarkable endurance strongly suggests that the story finds a special resonance in the collective unconscious.

Between the time when the early Greek anatomists studied the hearts of human subjects in Alexandria, Egypt, and the advent of the era when this organ began to be looked at in a radically new way—no longer as the focal node of emotions but as a muscular organ charged with propelling the blood—close to 1,900 years elapsed. William Harvey (1578–1657), with his discovery of the blood circulation, initiated this truly revolutionary conceptualization. The publication of his famous opus, the "Anatomical Exercises on the Movements of the Heart and the Blood in Animals" (*Exercitatio anatomica de motu cordis et sanguinis in animalibus*), commonly referred to as *De Motu Cordis*, did more than set the heart in a new light; it placed the whole of medicine on a new footing. The scientific method had arrived, and the heart would not be thought of in the same way as before.

The Seat of Passions Demystified and Tinkered With

Historians have pointedly remarked that the three greatest books of the English language were all written within a very short span of time in the 17th century, and at close intervals from each other.[10] These were the King James authorized version of the Bible (1611), the folio edition of Shakespeare's plays (1623) and Harvey's *De Motu Cordis* (1628). It has also been said that what the King James Bible was to the Church of England, and the Shakespearean folio to English letters, *De Motu Cordis* has been to medicine the world over. This praise is no exaggeration.

However, Harvey was very much a man of his time. Biographers commonly note that he was short, swarthy, mercurial, irascible, and carried with him a dagger, as did many men in his time, which he seemed inclined to reach for at the drop of a hat. It would be a mistake to think of him as a visionary possessed of a scientific spirit much ahead of the rest of his contemporaries, like Leonardo da Vinci. Apparently Harvey believed in witches: under the orders of King Charles I, he performed physical examinations of old women, looking for signs that would betray their demoniac condition. Had the telltale signs been present, the poor wretches might have died on the pyre, for such was the common fate at the time for those diagnosed with a diabolic connection. (Harvey's apologists are quick to point out that he never found inculpating evidence in the women he examined, and this they take to mean that he lent no credence to the existence of witches.) He also believed that a tumor of the breast had regressed after he had it stroked with the cold hand of a corpse.[11]

Like everyone in his time, he thought that the heart was, as he put it in *De Motu Cordis*, "the beginning of life, the Sun of the Microcosm, as proportionably the Sun deserves to be call'd the heart of the world." He believed its function was not merely the propulsion of the blood flow, but much more. It was the organ by which the blood "is perfected, made vegetable . . . defended from corruption . . ." In sum, its functions made the heart supreme in the organism, for "by nourishing, cherishing and vegetating, [the heart is] the foundation of life, and author of all."[12]

A man of the 17th century who called the heart, among other things, "the foundation of life," and the organ "from which all vigor and strength does flow," is apt to have believed that the heart was also the site where the sexual impulse originated. Harvey never said this, of course. But at least one modern commentator, Robert Erickson, has seen a more or less veiled yet unmistakable sexual imagery in the language that the illustrious physiologist used to describe his experiments and observations,. This is not without precedent. Other authors, precursors as well as contemporaries of William Harvey, represented the heart as a predominantly male organ—at least, the metaphors they used generally convey this signification. Thus, the first description of cardiac motions in *De Motu Cordis* is couched in wording that portrays the heart as *erectile*-contractile. During systole, wrote Harvey, this organ "is erected, and . . . it raises itself upwards into a point." And while it is contracting, says the modern exegete, Harvey's description is that of a "virtually phallic heart."[13] The same interpreter points out another passage where there appears to be a closer identification of the heart's ejected blood with an ejaculation of the male's generative organ, since the blood is identified with "the Sperm and prolifique Spirit of all living creatures."

In Aristotle's biology (and it must not be forgotten that Harvey was, to the last, a convinced Aristotelian), semen was a concoction or distillate—the ultimate refining derivative, so to speak—of the blood. The metaphoric language used in *De Motu Cordis*, by which the blood is depicted as life giving or life creating, and the heart as the organ that distributes its generative power to all parts of the organism (the body here figuratively represented as receptive, or "feminine"), may have suggested to the modern commentator a notion that he couches in striking words, namely that Harvey's heart is "unmistakably phallic—even masturbatory."[14]

Furthermore, Aristotle also notes that the heart is an organ with a distinct physiologic autonomy. In his treatise *On the Movement of Animals* (703b, 3-26), he insists that the heart is an organ with its own vitality; a bodily part that continues to beat independently for some time after all the other organs have died. Yet it is not the only organ endowed with this autonomy of function. For the ancients, the notion that the penis possesses independent life became commonplace: it enlarges and contracts on its own, and reason has very little power over its rebellious, wanton motions. It behaves, in the Aristotelian expression, like "a species of animal."

This is why two contemporary classical scholars, Giulia Sissa and Marcel Detienne, do not hesitate to affirm that the phallus and the heart incarnate the same life-giving power of Dionysus; in the cult of Dionysus, they share with wine a power manifested in gushing or outpouring.[15] But, they hasten to add, the Dionysian cult is not just a vulgar phallocracy: the male sex is not held to a place of higher importance than the female. The phallic representation in the pagan religion alludes to a life force that transcends human sexuality: the ineffable, vital energy that suffuses plants, animals, and all living beings—a puissance that is beyond either sex, even beyond our limited concept of sex or gender. If the votaries of Dionysus chose to represent this mighty force by a phallic symbol, we suspect that this is because in our species the generative organs happen to be more conspicuous in the male.

That the odd notion of a "phallic heart" exists in a larval state in the mind of some men is shown by an utterance that the 19th-century novelist Joris-Karl Huysmans (1848–1907) places in the mouth of a personage in his remarkable, decadent novel, *Là-Bas* (variously translated as *Down There* or *The Damned*): "The heart, reputedly the noble part of man, has the same shape as the penis, which is, so to speak, his vile part; this is very symbolic, for every love of the heart ends up in the part which it resembles."[16] From this curious statement, I gather that Huysmans may have been a great novelist but not much of an anatomist: he had rather fantastic notions of what a human heart looks like.

For thousands of years, cardiac symbolism was extended to cover God and man, the macrocosm and the microcosm of the body, sacred as well as profane love, the principle of life, the seat of passions, the foundation of our existence, and countless other meanings. Today the heart has been divorced from its manifold significations and reconceptualized as a mass of muscle; very complex and admirably well organized from a biologic standpoint, it is true, but in comparison with its former, astoundingly rich associations, the heart has suffered detriment. It is reduced, in essence, to a lump of flesh in charge of pumping the blood around the body.

This derogation was necessary in order to accommodate medicine's recent scientific and technological advances, especially cardiac transplants. The heart is no longer the principle of life. Modern technology has made it possible, with the use of respirators, to keep the heart of a patient beating for a very long time, even after he (or she) has entered a terminal phase of coma from which he will not recover. This time may be months or years—so long, as to cause a deterioration that will render the heart unfit for transplant. Hence, the need to change the concept of death. For centuries, a man was not "actually" dead until his heart stopped beating, his lungs stopped breathing, and his pulse ceased. But since the 1960s, this has changed in favor of "brain death," defined as irreversible coma and lack of responsiveness. This new definition was the work of an Ad Hoc Committee of the Harvard Medical School to Examine the Definition of Brain Death. Brain death did not exist before the 1960s, and the extraordinary significance of changing the age-old definition of death cannot escape even the least perceptive. This is one of the landmark changes that have occurred in human society, and it did not come about without trepidation.

Is a man whose heart is still beating "actually" dead? The moral, legal, and religious quandaries posed by this question are obvious and have been widely publicized. In 1968 a Japanese surgeon was charged with killing a patient for having removed his heart while it was still beating, in order to perform a cardiac transplant. Even though the patient was comatose, the court decided that the surgeon had not presented sufficient evidence to diagnose death. The charges were dropped in 1972, but, subsequently, cardiac transplants were banned in Japan and were not authorized until 1997, when brain death was officially recognized. Still, the Japanese are averse to this procedure, few people accept to be postmortem donors, and only 10 percent of those who need a cardiac transplant receive it in Japan—the rest must die or go abroad for the operation. In the United States, a distinguished cardiac surgeon, Richard Lower, was also accused of killing a patient in 1968, when he performed a cardiac transplant operation. The procedure was done shortly after the donor, a man who had sustained a serious head trauma, was declared dead, but without requesting permission from his surviving relatives. The surgeon was cleared of the charge four years later, when the new definition of death became acceptable to the courts.

The heart is no longer the supreme avatar of compassion, *caritas*, or unselfishness. Here too, transplants overturned this ancient belief. For it has always been assumed that to give your heart to someone else was an act of loving magnanimity and spiritual loftiness than which no greater could be imagined. Yet today hearts are exchanged in utterly anonymous and impersonal ways. Most often, the recipient does not know who the donor was, and vice versa. But even when the identities are known, the transcendent nature of the exchange seems diluted by the banality of the procedure. Yes: astounding as the reports of the first cardiac transplant in 1967 seemed to persons of my generation—no less momentous than the first landing on the moon, only two years later—the operation is now becoming a routine.

A conversation has been recorded between two patients who had exchanged a heart.[17] Patient A suffered from cystic fibrosis, a disease that had seriously damaged his lungs. The decision was made to treat him with a cadaveric transplant of heart and lungs. His own heart went to patient B, whose heart had been damaged beyond repair by a disease of unknown origin involving the cardiac muscle. Patients A and B were attending a clinic to monitor their posttransplant clinical progress, when they entered into a conversation and fortuitously found out that they were the subjects of the exchange. This accidental discovery brought forth no stupefaction

on either side; there was no mind-boggling wonderment, no be-
dazzled exclamations of "You have my heart!" or "Your heart beats
inside my chest!" All there was could be described as a polite well-
wishing. Both patients were very happy that they had survived and
that they seemed to be recovering from the operation. And perhaps
this relatively muted response was all that was warranted. For what
grounds had A to claim ownership of a heart now integrated in
another organism? Or B to think that a heart on which his life now
depended was less his own?

All this is a far cry from the heart as "the ultimate symbol of
human affection."

The heart is no longer the seat of love. After the first human-
to-human heart transplant was performed in South Africa on
December 3, 1967, by the dashing, highly "mediatic" young surgeon Christian Barnaard, a veritable torrent of troubling questions
came to the fore. Not the least of these came from the lay public,
unaccustomed to seeing an organ charged with age-old symbolisms
suddenly reduced to the status of mere mechanical contraption.
The patient who received the heart transplant, Louis Washkansky,
was projected to international fame as much as his surgeon: this
was probably one of the most highly publicized surgical operations
in the history of the world. The questions posed by the crowd
of journalists brought into relief the general apprehension with
which the people regarded this unprecedented tampering with a
most mysterious and enigmatic bodily organ. Asked about her reaction to her husband's operation, Mrs. Washkansky declared that
she had been afraid that, upon recovering from the anesthesia, her
spouse would no longer love her: "Like everyone else, I thought the
heart controls all your emotions and your personality," she said.[18]

The heart is no longer the sacred core of one's being. Journalists asked a recovering Mr. Washkansky in his hospital room, which they crowded (an intrusion of a kind that would be inconceivable today), what it felt like for him, a Jew, to carry in his chest the beating heart of a Gentile. I am not aware of his reply, but it is unlikely to have been too profound, since his clinical condition precluded any serious mental pondering; he died on the 18th postoperative day. Yet the question of the heart's rapport with personal identity had been very much present in the field of transplant surgery. It was with all deliberation that Christian Barnaard avoided, in his pioneering operation, the transfer of a heart between patients of different races. In a country that still adhered to apartheid, the least that could be said is that this avoidance was eminently prudent.

In his second operation, though, Barnaard used a "colored" man named Clive Haupt as donor and a white man, Philip Blaiberg, as recipient. The biologic mechanism of rejection—that is, the failure of the engrafted organ "to take" inside its new host—was incompletely understood, and the lack of effective ways to combat it was the main cause of death of most patients operated on in the late 1960s. However, Mr. Blaiberg managed to survive for 19 months. This gave occasion for newspaper editorialists to comment, with no small dose of sarcasm, about the quandaries created by a white man with a black man's heart in a country ruled by racist, discriminatory policies. If a white man is allowed to use a dead black man's heart, does it follow that the two should be allowed, when living, to sit together in all the public places from which blacks are generally excluded? To this rhetorical question, the answer was "probably not." As to the surgeon who produced this admixture, this chimera, "he should know that he faces serious charges." Moreover, wrote one editorialist, "there is no provision in the Group Areas Act for black hearts to beat in white neighborhoods." And the sardonic commentary ends with the conclusion that Mr. Haupt was guilty of posthumously infringing the law.[19]

However, thousands of years of symbolism, myth, legend, and deeply ingrained metaphor cannot be brushed aside so casually. Is it really true that the heart is no longer the center and pivot of the physical person? We still feel it ticking in what is, to most of us, the center of our physical person. Do we really believe in the new definition of death? Important as it is to accept it for the sake of orderly social life and the progress of medicine, deep inside we still feel that the moment our heart stops beating will mark the time when the jaws of death trap us to begin their work of grinding and trituration. Will lovers stop representing their longing as their heart's ache? Will parents laid low by the ingratitude of their children not speak of its ultimate breakage? Not likely.

Nor is it true that science reduces the heart to a mere propelling pump, one more mechanical device in its dehumanizing conception of man as machine, "protoplasmic robot," or "flesh manikin." Medicine rose to the status of science only when it began to anatomize—that is, to sever, or separate. For the immense complexity of the body was such that it could not be understood, except by studying its parts one by one, each one separately and in isolation. Thus, Western medicine was built upon a model of organ independence and functional autonomy: the gastrointestinal system is good to digest the food, and nothing else; the optical system is free from any service, save that of seeing; audition is equally sovereign and enfranchised with respect to any other bodily function apart from hearing; and so on. But as medical science advances, it realizes that the interrelations between seemingly separate organs and systems are greater than at first suspected.

Colors do not look quite the same when seen while listening to soothing and to stimulating music: audition influences eyesight. Objects seem colder in blue than in red: vision influences tactile perception. The intestines are seeded with neuroendocrine cells that make the intestine an endocrine organ existing in "dispersed state" and an integral part of the nervous system. Abundant scattered groups of neuroendocrine cells, the existence of which is only now beginning to be widely recognized, also exist in the lungs.[20] Perhaps even the thinking function, traditionally the exclusive domain of the brain, may admit of some sharing, however limited, with other organs. Friedrich Nietzsche, the German philosopher, was of the opinion that we think with our whole body: our bones, our viscera, and our skin. For him the brain was a mere "apparatus for concentration" of thought. His was a vivid formulation of the "knowing from the heart," to which I referred earlier. We may deem this opinion fanciful, but it is a fact that the sundering biomedical model is increasingly perceived as insufficient, and the unitary or holistic concept, long held in high esteem in Eastern world cultures, grows in importance.

In chapter XLVII, part II of Miguel de Cervantes's *Don Quixote*, the mad knight's rotund squire, Sancho Panza, has been duped into believing that he is governor of an (illusory) island. A fake personal physician tortures him by stopping him from eating every plate placed tantalizingly before him, until the good squire is beside himself. At that moment, he is warned that spies are coming to assassinate him and is told to summon all his courage. Would he strengthen his heart, the traditional seat of bravery? All that Sancho wants is to eat. Therefore, in his usual earthy style, he voices the trite reality of our nature: "If we are to be ready for those battles that menace us, then we must be well fed, because *it is the tripes that carry the heart, not the heart the tripes . . .*"

Idealize as we might our bodily organs, the incontestable reality will impose itself in the end. There are no hierarchies in the body's component parts. The body is one, its cogs and wheels inextricably interdependent. The heart, for all the nobility and bravery that our fancy adorns it with, will be nothing without the tripes that are carrying it.

The heart is currently the subject of a more subtle holistic reassessment. Contrary to popular wisdom, the medical profession long refused to see in the heart the "shock organ" of tumultuous emotions. A very strong emotion can negatively affect health: multisecular experience teaches that. Yet doctors maintained that the heart was only secondarily affected by what the ancients called "the passions." If collapse occurred following emotional shock, the real cause was thought to be age, arteriosclerosis, antecedent cardiac lesions, or pathology elsewhere in the body; emotional turmoil was merely the precipitating accident, the drop that caused the cup to overflow. That panic, sudden fright, a major surprise, disillusionment, or overwhelming moral distress could cause stoppage of the heart—and that this could be irreversible—was thought to be a groundless notion of the laity, a quaint popular belief without scientific backing. That a perfectly healthy lover just ditched by his paramour should suddenly fall to the ground, pale and pulseless; or that one who just discovered the traitorousness of his love-object should clutch his left chest with a tense hand and fall instantaneously, as if fulminated—these scenes were thought to belong in dramatic compositions and theatrical performances, not in clinical descriptions pretending to scientific validity and vouched by cardiologists.

However, the opinion of the profession is changing. The mutual rapport between mental states and cardiac activity is currently originating talk of "heart-brain medicine" in medical circles.[21] Cardiac lesions are demonstrable in those who die while under great mental stress,[22] even when no other internal lesions are found, as in the case of persons who see themselves as victims of a curse, voodoo, or black magic.[23] Similar devastation of the heart occurs in perfectly healthy people who find themselves in the midst of a war or an earthquake or other natural disaster, even when they sustain no physical traumas. Support for the concept of heart-brain medicine is afforded by the evolving knowledge of the rich innervation of the heart. Neurons of various types exist in ganglia extrinsic to the heart as well as intrinsic to it; they form a neuronal system so complex in its ramifications, its interrelationships, and its connections to the central nervous system, that it is no wonder that an investigator has called this system "the little brain on the heart."[24]

Most importantly, to the cardiac lesions associated with emotional stress, which pathologists have known for some time, is being added a clinical picture appropriately supported by modern diagnostic technology. This condition has been described under the graphic name of "the broken heart syndrome."[25] The patients are free from coronary atherosclerosis, yet following a traumatic emotional episode, they complain of chest pain, manifest some electrocardiographic abnormalities, and have a very mild elevation of cardiac enzymes. The most distinctive feature is a unique pattern of abnormal contractility of the left ventricle. The tip of the heart and its middle portion contract feebly or not at all. As a consequence, when the heart is visualized radiographically by means of contrast media, its silhouette is distorted, appearing crushed, pressed, or strangulated. Typically, the patients recover promptly, but some may die. A person with a broken heart is, indeed, crushed by a weight higher than he, or she, can bear.[26]

I was always intrigued by the peculiar cardiac pathology of patients who die under the circumstances mentioned. Unlike myocardial infarction, where the cardiac muscle dies within a well-defined region of the heart (corresponding to the area supplied by a coronary artery), in the broken heart syndrome the damage is patchy: a focus of necrosis here or of dissolution of cardiac fibers there, randomly distributed. It is hard to suppress the thought that the heart has been shattered in pieces. Perhaps the imagination of the poets has been prescient. John Donne (1572–1631), mystical English poet, complained that love's disappointment had rudely treated his heart: "At one first blow did shiver it as glass." He did not die of the blow but carried with him a broken heart:

> Therefore I think my breast hath all
> Those pieces still, though they be not unite;
> And now as broken glasses show
> A hundred lesser faces, so
> My rags of heart can like, wish and adore,
> But after one such love, can love no more.

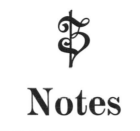

Notes

Digestive

1. For a learned discussion of the centrality of the stomach in ancient medical thought, see Walter Pagel: *The Smiling Spleen: Paracelsianism in Storm and Stress*. New York: Karger, 1984, pp. 119–129.

2. Ibid, pg. 124.

3. Roy Porter. *The Greatest Benefit to Mankind: A Medical History of Humanity*. New York: W. W. Norton, 1997, pg. 102.

4. L. Testut and A. Latarjet. *Traité d'Anatomie Humaine*, 9th edition. Paris: G. Doin & Co., 1949. (The quoted description is author's translation.)

5.   Robert E. Grant. *Lectures on Comparative Anatomy: Delivered in the University of London during 1833.* Published in *The Lancet* for 1833–1834, pg. 738.

6.   Ibid, pg. 787.

7.   For a review of past theories of gastric digestion up to the 19th century, see: John R. Young: *An Experimental Inquiry into the Principles of Nutrition and the Digestive Process* (reprint from 1803 edition). Urbana-Champaign, Ill.: Board of Trustees of the University of Illinois, 1959. See, in particular, the helpful preface by William C. Rose.

8.   Lazzaro Spallanzani. *La Digestion Stomacale: De la Digestion des Animaux à Estomac Membraneux.* Paris: G. Masson, 1893, pg. 29 (reprint of a work that first appeared in 1783; Geneva, Jean Senebier). The quoted paragraphs from this source are the author's translations.

9.   Ibid, pg. 106.

10. Ibid, pg. 107 cf.

11. Felice Grondona. "Des expériments de Lazzaro Spallanzani sur la digestion aux applications thérapeutiques du suc gastrique." *Clio Medica* 8 (4) (1973): 285–294. This article contains a rich bibliography, chiefly of Italian primary sources, on the therapeutic use of gastric juice.

12. Jerome J. Bylebyl. "William Beaumont, Robley Dunglison, and the 'Philadelphia Physiologists.'" *Journal of the History of Medicine and Allied Sciences* 25 (1) (1970): 3–21.

13. Horace W. Davenport. "What happened to the third bottle of St. Martin's gastric juice?" *Physiologist* 21 (3) (1978): 35–39. May be consulted online at: *www.the-aps.org/publications/tphys/legacy/1978/ issue3/35.pdf* (site visited on April 11, 2007).

14. William Beaumont. *Experiments and Observations on the Gastric Juice and the Physiology of Digestion.* Plattsburgh, New York: F. P. Allen, 1833.

15. Joseph Szurszewski. "Motions of Alexis St. Martin's Stomach." *Federation Proceedings* 44 (November 1985): 2894–2896.

16. Quoted by Robert Helms. "Alexis St. Martin (1794–1880): The Intrepid Guinea Pig of the Great Lakes." Consulted online at: *www.guineapigzero.com/AlexisStMartin.html* (site visited on April 13, 2007).

17. Ibid.

18. Ronald Numbers and William Orr. "William Beaumont's reception at home and abroad." *Isis* 72 (264) (December 1981): 590–612.

Scatology

1. François Rabelais. *Le Tiers Livre* (chapter 15 in *Oeuvres Complètes*). Paris: Seuil, 1973, pg. 425 (author's translation).

2. Quoted by Claude Gaignebet and Marie Claude Perier. *L'Homme et l'excretum. De l'excreté à l'exécré.* In: *Histoire des Moeurs.* Vol. 1 Encyclopédie de la Pléiade. Paris: Gallimard, 1991, pp. 831–839.

3. See: *The Sayings of Chuang-tzu: A New Translation by James Ware.* Taiwan: Confucius Publishing Company, undated (bilingual edition), pg. 268. Also: *The Texts of Taoism: The Sacred Books of China translated by James Legge* (in two volumes). The Writings of Chuang Tzu, part II, vol. 2. New York: Dover Publications, 1962 (first published by Oxford University Press in 1891), pp. 66–67; and *Les Philosophes Taoistes.* Gallimard, 1969, pp. 254–255.

4. *www.godchecker.com/pantheon/chinese-mythology.php?deity=ZI-GU* (site visited on August 8, 2006).

5. The significance of excrement in ancient Mesoamerican civilizations is explored in: Cecelia F. Klein: "Teocuitlatl, 'Divine Excrement': the significance of 'holy shit' in ancient Mexico," special issue on scatological art, Gabriel Weisberg, guest editor. *Art Journal* 52 (3) (1993): 20–27. See especially, for an interesting treatment of this topic: Alfredo López Austin: *Vieja Historia de la Mierda*. Mexico City: Edíciones, Toledo, 1988.

6. François Rabelais, loc. cit.: *Gargantua*, chapter 40.

7. Pliny. *Natural History*, Book XV, xxxvi, 120, translated by H. Rackham. Cambridge, Mass.: Harvard University Press, Loeb Classical Library (1986, last reprint), pg. 369.

8. Quoted by Jacques-Antoine Dulaure. *Des Divinités Génératrices chez les Anciens et les Modernes*. Paris: A. Van Genep; Société du Mercure de France, 1905.

9. Herodotus. *The Histories*, Book II, 75–77, translated by Aubrey de Sélincourt. New York: Penguin Books, 1972, pg. 158.

10. Diodorus Siculus. *Library of History*, Book I, 81, translated by C. H. Oldfather. Cambridge, Mass.: Harvard University Press, Loeb Classical Library, 1989, pg. 281.

11. Bruno Haliqua and Bernand Ziskind. *Medicine in the Days of the Pharaohs*, translated by M. B. De Bevoise, with a foreword by Donald B. Redford. Cambridge, Mass.: The Belknap Press of Harvard University Press, 2005, pp. 13–14.

12. L. Viso, J. Uriach, et al. "The 'Guardians of the anus' and their practice." *International Journal of Colorectal Diseases* 10 (1995): 229–231.

13. P. Defosses and A. Martinet. "Le Lavement." *Presse Médicale*. Vol. 1, 1903, pp. 309–315.

14. This work was translated into French (by an unnamed transl) under the name of *L'Instrument de Molière*. Paris: Damascene Morgand and Charles Fatout, 1878.

15. Élie Metchnikoff. *The Prolongation of Life: Optimistic Studies*. New York: G. P. Putnam's Sons, 1908. See also: Scott H. Podolsky. "Cultural Divergence: Élie Metchnikoff's Bacillus bulgaricus therapy and his underlying concept of health." *Bulletin of the History of Medicine* 72 (1) (1988): 1–27.

16. S. Jonas. *Cent Portraits de Médecins Illustres*. Paris: Academia S. P. R. L. Masson, 1960, pg. 223.

17. Christopher Lawrence: "Medical Minds, Surgical Bodies: Corporeality and the Doctors." Chapter 5 in: Christopher Lawrence and Steven Chapin (editors): *Science Incarnate: Historical Embodiments of Natural Knowledge*. Chicago: University of Chicago Press, 1998, pp. 156–201.

18. Richard Gordon. *The Alarming History of Medicine: Amusing Anecdotes from Hippocrates to Heart Transplants*. New York: St. Martin's Press, 1993.

19. J. Lacey Smith. "Sir Arbuthnot Lane, Chronic Intestinal Stasis, and Autointoxication." *Annals of Internal Medicine* 96 (1992): 365–369.

20. A rich source of bibliography on Arbuthnot Lane's life and work is the thorough monographic work of Ann Daly: "Fantasy surgery, 1880–1930; with special reference to Sir William Arbuthnot Lane." *Clio Medica* 38 (1996): 1–359.

21. For the orthopedic work of Sir Arbuthnot Lane, see: C. C. Jeffrey: "A fracture plated by Sir William Arbuthnot Lane in 1912." *Journal of Bone and Joint Surgery* 41-B (British volume) (2) (May 1959):

368–369; and A. R. Jones: "Sir William Arbuthnot Lane." *Journal of Bone and Joint Surgery* 34-B (British volume) (3) (1952): 478–482.

22. Robert Bell. "Constipation viewed as a disease per se and as an exciting cause of disease." *Lancet* 1 (1880): 243–234; 282–285.

23. Seton S. Pringle. "An address on chronic intestinal stasis." *British Medical Journal* I (1914): 183–188.

24. Arthur J. Brock. "Autointoxication and subinfection." *British Medical Journal* I (1914): 273. See also J. G. Adami: "Chronic intestinal stasis: autointoxication and subinfection." Ibid, pp. 177–183.

25. E. Barclay-Smith. "A case of extreme visceral dislocation: with remarks on the functional interpretation of agminated glands of the intestine." *Proceedings of the Cambridge Philosophical Society* 12 (1903): 18–26.

26. Quoted by Ann Daly, loc. cit. See reference 20, above.

27. Sir William Arbuthnot Lane expounded on the characteristics of his patients and the main features of their clinical picture at the respected Royal Society of Medicine in London, during a meeting that comprised six sessions between March 10 and May 7, 1913. The proceedings were published in *Proceedings of the Royal Society of Medicine* 6 (1913). See his presentation entitled "Alimentary Toxaemia: Its Sources, Consequences and Treatment." The quotation is from page 102.

28. Ibid, pg. 108.

29. Ibid. See appendix, with a letter from Sir Arbuthnot Lane, pg. 350.

30. W. C. Alvarez. "Origin of the so-called autointoxication symptoms." *Journal of the American Medical Association* 72 (1919): 8–13. See also: A. N. Donaldson. "Relation of constipation to intestinal intoxication." *Journal of the American Medical Association* 78 (1922): 884–888.

31. W. E. Tanner. *Sir William Arbuthnot Lane, Bart: His Life and Work.* London: Baillière, Tindall & Cox, 1946.

32. Thomas S. N. Chen and Peter S. Y. Chen. "Intestinal autointoxication: A Medical Leitmotif." *Journal of Clinical Gastroenterology* 11 (4) (1989): 434–441.

Respiratory

1. *Les Cyniques Grecs: Fragments et témoignages.* Libraire Générale Française, 1992, pg. 101 (author's translation).

2. MacDonald Critchley. 'Sleepy Sickness.' Curious chapter of medical history." *Medical and Health Annual.* Chicago: Encyclopaedia Britannica, 1992, pg. 212.

3. W. A. Tossach. "A man dead in appearance recovered by distending the lungs with air." The *Medical Essays and Observations* V (part 2). Edinburgh: Philosophical Society of Edinburgh, 1744, pp. 605–608.

4. P. Safar. "History of cardiopulmonary-cerebral resuscitation." In: W. Kaye, N. G. Bircher, editors. "Cardiopulmonary resuscitation." *Clinical Critical Care Medicine* 16 (1989): 1–53.

5. R. V. Trubuhovich. "History of mouth-to-mouth rescue breathing, part 1." *Critical Care and Resuscitation* 7 (2005): 250–257.

6. A. Barrington Baker. "Artificial respiration, the history of an idea." *Medical History* XV (4) (October 1971): 336–351.

7. Z. Rosen and J. T. Davidson. "Respiratory resuscitation in ancient Hebrew sources." *Anaesthesia and Analgesia* 51 (1972): 502–505.

8. Quoted in: Alfred Franklin. *La Vie Privée d'Autrefois.* In 2 volumes. Vol. I: *L'Enfant. La Naissance, Le Baptême.* Paris: Plon, Nourrit et Co., 1895, pp. 71–72.

9. Paulus Bagellardus. *Libellus de aegritudinibus infantum*. Barval, 1472, pg. 3. Quoted by Barrington Baker; note 6 above.

10. From a note appearing in the English periodical *Jopson's Coventry Mercury* on May 31, 1784. Quoted by Roy Porter in: *Flesh in the Age of Reason*. New York: W. W. Norton, 2003.

11. P. Defosses and A. Martinet. "Le Lavement." *La Presse Médicale* 1 (1903): 311.

12. J. Trevor Hughes. "Miraculous deliverance of Anne Green: an Oxford case of resuscitation in the seventeenth century." *British Medical Journal* 285 (1982): 1792–1793.

13. W. K. C. Guthrie. *A History of Greek Philosophy, Vol. 1: The Early Presocratics and the Pythagoreans*. Cambridge, Mass.: Cambridge University Press, 1962, pg. 127.

14. Francis Bacon. *Historia Vitae et Mortis*. In: James Spedding, Robert Leslie Ellis, and Douglas Denon Heath (editors). *The Works of Francis Bacon, Baron of Verulam, Viscount of Alban and Lord High Chancellor of England*, Vol. 5. London: Longman and Co., 1858, pg. 312.

15. Plutarch. *Table Talk*. In: *Moralia*: Book VIII, chapter I, 697–700. (In 16 vols.) See Vol. 9, translated by Edwin L. Minar Jr., F. H. Sandbach, and W. C. Helmond. Cambridge, Mass.: Loeb Classical Library, Harvard University Press, 1961, reprinted 1969, pp. 7–21.

16. John Mayow. *Medico-Physical Works, being a translation of Tractatus Quinque Medico-Physici*. 1674. Edinburgh: A.C.D.L.B. Alembic Club, 1907, pp. 202–204. (A re-edition was published in 1957.)

17. Kenneth D. Keele. "Physiology." In: Allen G. Debus (editor): *Medicine in Seventeenth Century England*. Berkeley, Calif.: University of California Press, 1974, pp. 147–181.

18. Francis Chinard. Priestley and Lavoisier: Oxygen and Carbon Dioxide. Chapter 12 in: Donald F. Proctor (editor): *A History of Breathing Physiology*. New York: Marcel Dekker, 1995, pp. 203–222. The latter work is an excellent source of information on the study of breathing from antiquity to the modern age.

19. Luigi Pirandello. *Soffio* (author's translation). In: *L'Illustre Estinto e Altre Novelle*. Biblioteca Ideale Tascabile. Milan: Opportunity Books, 1995, pp. 49–58.

20. Quotations from the correspondence of Chopin and George Sand in this chapter were taken from Jean-José Boutaric. *Laënnec, Balzac, Chopin et le stéthoscope ou la diffusion de l'auscultation médiate durant la première moitié du XIX siècle*. Paris: Glyphe et Biotem, 2004 (author's translations).

21. Maria Gondolo della Riva Masera. *Chopin. Scorci Biografici*. Turin: L'Arciere, 1989, pp. 143–144.

22. Jean-José Boutaric, loc. cit. See note 20.

23. Lu Hsun. *Medicine*. In: *Selected Works of Lu Hsun* (in 4 vols.). Peking: Foreign Languages Press, 1966, Vol. 1, pp. 29–39.

24. René-Théophile-Hyacinthe Laënnec. *De l'Auscultation Médiate, ou traité du diagnostic des maladies des poumons et du coeur, fondé principalement sur ce nouveau moyen d'exploration*. Paris: J. A. Brosson & J. S. Chaudé, 1819. See part III, chapter 1, entitled *Exploration du Râle*, pp. 2–9.

25. Ibid, pp. 2–5.

26. Fernando del Paso. *Palinuro de México*. In: *Obras*, Vol. 1. El Colegio Nacional & Fondo de Cultura Económica. Mexico City, 2000, pg. 936 ff. This novel exists in English translation as *Palinuro of Mexico*, translated by Elizabeth Plaister, Dalkey Archives Press, 1996.

27. For a learned and perceptive exploration of the symbolic meanings in the alluded text of Chuang-tzu, see: François Billeter. *Études Sur Tchouang-tseu.* Paris: Editions Allia, 2004, pp. 117–159. As is usual in translations from the Chinese, various Western language versions differ substantially among themselves, even though they refer to the same original text. In this case, I am referring to Book 2, part 1 of Chuang-tzu's complete works, for which we consulted the following versions: *The Texts of Taoism,* translated by James Legge (in 2 vols.). New York: Dover Publications, 1962 (reprint of edition first published by Oxford University Press in 1891), pp. 176–202; *Philosophes Taoistes.* French translation and annotations by Liou Kwa-Hway and Benedykt Grynpas. Paris: Gallimard, Collection Pléiade, 1969, pp. 93–104; *The Sayings of Chuang Tzu. A New Translation by James Ware.* Taiwan: Confucius Publishing Co., undated, pg. 12.

Reproductive

Part I: Female

1. Soranus. *Gynecology,* Book I, 9. Translated by Owsei Temkin. Baltimore: Johns Hopkins University Press, 1956, pg. 10.
2. Hippocrates. *Generation* 9–10, 1. In: *Oeuvres complètes d'Hippocrate: traduction nouvelle avec le texte grec en regard.* Translated by E. Littré (10 vols.). Paris: Baillière, 1839–1861, pp. 628–629. All references to Hippocrates are from this edition unless otherwise stated. Hereinafter referred to as Littré.
3. Publius Cornelius Tacitus. "The Fall of Agrippina." Chapter 11 in: *The Annals of Imperial Rome.* Translated by Michael Grant.

New York: Penguin Books, 1983 (first published in 1956), pp. 284–319.

4. Soranus, loc. cit. Book I, pp. 10–11.

5. Aristotle. *Generation of Animals*, Book II, vii, 20, 746ª.

6. F. Kuldien. "The seven cells of the uterus: the doctrine and its roots." *Bulletin of the History of Medicine* 39 (5) (1965): 415–423.

7. Pliny. *Natural History*, Book VII, iii, 33. (In 10 vols.) Translated by H. Rackham. Cambridge, Mass.: Loeb Classical Library, Harvard University Press, 1989 (first published in 1942).

8. Quoted by F. Kuldien, see 6 above, and, by the same author: "The legal aspect of the doctrine of the seven uterine cells," *Bulletin of the History of Medicine* 40 (6) (1966): 544–546.

9. *Aerétée. Signes et causes des maladies aiguës* 2.11 Translated by R. T. H. Laënnec, edited and with comments by Miko D. Grmek. Geneva: Droz, 2000, pp. 61–62.

10. L. Testut and O. Jacob. *Tratado de anatomía topográfica con aplicaciones médico-quirúrgicas.* (2 vols.) 8th edition, Vol. 2. Mexico: Salvat, 1952, pg. 516.

11. Natalie Angier. *Woman: An Intimate Geography.* New York: Anchor Books, 2000, pp. 101–102.

12. Véronique Dasen. "Métamorphoses de l'utérus d'Hippocrate à Ambroise Paré." *Gesnerus* Vol. 59, 2002, pp. 167–186.

13. Littré VIII (*Morbus Mulieris*) 1.78: pp. 174–175, and 2.135: pp. 308–309.

14. Véronique Dasen, loc. cit., note 12 above.

15. Jean-Pierre Vernant. *Au miroir de Méduse.* Chapter VI in: *L'Individu, la mort, l'amour. Soi-même et l'autre en Grèce ancienne.* Paris: Gallimard, 1989, pp. 117–129.

16. Pausanias. *Description of Greece*. (6 vols.) Vol. 1. Translated by W. H. S. Jones. Book II, xxi, 4-6. London: Heinemann, 1918, pg. 359.

17. Aristotle. *On Dreams*. 2, 25, 460a. In: *The Complete Works of Aristotle* (in 2 vols.). The revised Oxford translation, edited by Jonathan Barnes. Vol. 1 Princeton University Press, 6th printing, 1995: pg. 731.

18. Pliny. *Natural History*. (In 10 vols.) Book VII, xv, 64–xvi. Translated by H. Rackham. Cambridge, Mass.: Loeb Classical Library, Harvard University Press, 1989, Vol. 2, pg. 549.

19. Cesare Lombroso. *La Donna Delinquente*, 3rd Edition. Turin: Fratelli Bocca, 1915, pg. 96.

20. Camile Paglia. *Sexual Personae: Art and Decadence from Nefertiti to Emily Dickinson*. New York: Vintage Books, 1991, pg. 11.

21. Ibid.

22. Natalie Angier, loc. cit., pg. 107.

23. Karen Houppert. "The Final Period." Op-ed contributor to the *New York Times*, July 17, 2007.

24. Margie Profet. "Menstruation as a defense against pathogens transported by sperm." *Quarterly Review of Biology* 68 (1993): pp. 335–386.

25. Beverly I. Strassman. "The evolution of endometrial cycles and menstruation." *Quarterly Review of Biology* 71 (1996): 181–220.

26. H. E. Skipper and S. Perry. "Kinetics of normal and leukemic leukocyte populations and relevance to chemotherapy." *Cancer Research* 30 (1970): 1883–1897.

27. Guido Majno and Isabelle Joris. *Cells, Tissues, and Disease: Principles of General Pathology* (2nd edition). Cambridge, Mass.: Blackwell Science, 2004, pp. 200–219.

28. Ibid, pg. 219.

29. An English language version of Thomas Mann's novella appeared under the title of *The Black Swan*, translated from the German by Willard R. Trask. Berkeley, Calif.: University of California Press, 1990. (The first English language version of the novella was published by Alfred Knopf, New York, 1954.)

Part II: Male

30. Katharine Park. *Secrets of Women: Gender, Generation, and the Origin of Human Dissection*. New York: Zone Books, 2006. See, especially, chapter 2: "Secrets of Women," pp. 77–120.

31. E. S. Pretorius, E. S. Siegelman, P. Ramchandani, et al. "MR Imaging of the penis." *Radiographic* 21 (2001): S283–S299.

32. Diane A. Kelly. "Penises are variable-volume hydrostatic skeletons." *Annals of the New York Academy of Sciences* 1101 (2007): 453–463.

33. B. A. Ng, R. G. Ramsey, and J. P. Corey. "The distribution of nasal erectile mucosa as visualized by magnetic resonance." *Ear, Nose and Throat Journal* 78 (3) (1999): 163–366.

34. On the role of Wilhelm Fliess in psychiatry, see: H. P. Blum. "Freud, Fliess and the parenthood of psychoanalysis." *Psychoanalytical Quarterly* 59 (1) (1990): 21–40. Fleiss's major opus initially appeared in 1897 but was more recently published in French translation. See: Wilhelm Fliess: *Les relations entre le nez et les organes génitaux de la femme*. Translated from the German by P. Auch and J. Guir. Paris: Le Seuil, 1977.

35. J. M. Masson (editor). *The Complete Letters of Sigmund Freud to Wilhelm Fliess 1887–1904*. Cambridge, Mass.: Harvard University Press, 1985, pp. 45–49.

36. B. Mautner. "Freud's 'lost' dream and the schism with Wilhelm Fliess." *International Journal of Psycho-Analysis* 75 (pt. 2) (April 1994): 321–333. See also: B. Mautner: "Freud's Irma dream: a psychoanalytical interpretation." Ibid, 72 (pt. 2) (1991): 275–286; and Comment, in: Ibid, 74 (pt. 1) (February 1993): 179–180.

37. The biographical information on François de la Peyronie comes from the two-part monograph written by Professor E. Forgue and published in the now disappeared monthly magazine *Les Biographies Médicales: Notes por servir à l'histoire de la médecine et ses grands médecins.* Vol. 10, Nos. 5 (June–July): 291–304, and 6 (Aug.–Sept.): 305–320; 1936. (Paris, Baillière.)

38. Quoted by E. Forgue. Ibid, part I, pp. 303–304.

39. The original communication by la Peyronie on the disease that bears his name appeared as *Mémoire sur quelques obstacles qui s'opposent à l'éjaculation naturelle de la semence.* It was published in *Mémoires de l'Académie Royale de Chirurgie,* Vol. 1 (no. 4); 1743, pp. 425–434. The main focus of this article is the difficulty in ejaculation secondary to the presence of the abnormal indurations. Semen, writes la Peyronie, is ejaculated retrogradely; in other words, to the bladder instead of to the outside, because the abnormal hardened tissue opposes an obstacle to its normal physiologic course. (The quoted paragraphs are the author's translations.)

40. Ibid, pp. 431–432.

41. Gustave Lenotre. *Napoléon: Croquis de l'Epopée.* Paris: Bernard Grasset, 1932, pp. 221–222.

42. Ibid, pg. 225.

43. A recent review of the theories on Napoléon's cause of death is: Alessandro Lugli, Inti Zlobec, Gad Singer, Andrea Kopp Lugli,

Luigi M. Terracciano, and Robert M. Genta: "Napoléon Bonaparte's Gastric Cancer: A clinicopathologic approach to staging, pathogenesis and etiology." *Nature Clinical Practice of Gastroenterology and Hepatology* 4 (1) (2007): 52–57. This reference contains a rich bibliography that will be helpful to all those interested in researching Napoléon's end. This article was posted on the Internet in January 2007. See: *www.medscape.com/viewarticle/550333_1*

44. Louis-Etienne St.-Denis. *Souvenirs du Mameluck Ali sur l'Empereur Napoléon*. Paris: P. Payot, 1926.

45. Judith Pascoe. "Collect-Me-Nots." Article published in the *New York Times*, May 17, 2007.

46. Quoted in: Marc Bonnard and Michel Schouman. *Histoires du Pénis*. Paris: Editions du Rocher, 1999, pp. 101–105. These authors reproduce the auction house's catalogue page with the description of lot number 54.

47. Ibid, pp. 104–105.

48. Stanley M. Bierman. "The peripatetic posthumous peregrination of Napoléon's penis." *Journal of Sex Research* 29 (4) (1992): 579.

49. Charles Hamilton. *Auction Madness*. New York: Everett House Publishers, 1981.

50. Quoted on several websites on the Internet that devote attention to the strange item in the St. Petersburg's Erotica Museum: *www. themight yorgan.com/features_rasputin.html*; *www.st-petersburg-life.com/st-petersburg/rasputins-penis*. On its possible false nature, see *www.museumofhoaxes.com/hoax/weblog/comments/1162*.

51. The Timewatch documentary, entitled "Who Killed Rasputin?" is described online at: *www.bbc.co.uk/print/pressoffice/pressreleases/stories/2004/09_september19/rasputin.shtml*. Site visited on August 10, 2007.

52. David Friedman. *A Mind of Its Own: A Cultural History of the Penis.* New York: The Free Press, 2001. Friedman's book is a serious and very comprehensive research on many aspects of the theme described in its subtitle. For penile measurements, see chapter 3, entitled "The Measuring Stick," pp. 103–147.

53. J. A. S. Collin de Plancy. *Dictionnaire critique des reliques et des images miraculeuses*, Vol. II. Paris: Guien et Cie, 1824, pg. 47.

54. O. Augustus Wall. *Sex and Sex Worship.* St. Louis, Mo.: C. V. Mosby, 1919. Quoted by Marc Bonnard and Michel Schouman: *Histoires du Pénis* (see note 44).

55. J. A. S. Collin de Plancy. Ibid.

56. Donato Calvi de Bergamo. *Propinomio Evangélico o Evangélicas Resoluciones. En las cuales con el fundamento de las Divinas Escrituras, Santos Padres Históricos I Expositores se demuestra claramente quienes fueron algunos personages, i sugetos, de quienes se hace mencion en los Evangelios, sin expressar sus nombres, con otras particularidades dignas de saberse.* (Spanish translation by Juan Joseph Gherzi de la Fuente). Printed in Seville, 1733.

57. Johan Huizinga. *The Waning of the Middle Ages.* Mineola, N.Y.: Dover Publications, 1999 (reprinted from the 1924 English language edition published by Edward Arnold & Co.), pg. 1.

Cardiovascular

1. Blaise Pascal. *Oeuvres Complètes.* Paris: Seuil, 1963. *Pensées* Nos. 423–424 (or 277–278 in the Brunschvig edition).

2. We used the edition of J. A. Smith and W. D. Ross of *The Works of Aristotle.* See Vol. V: *De Generatione Animalium*, translated by Arthur Platt. Oxford: Clarendon Press, 1958 (reprinted from first edition, 1912).

3. The Latin text of the critical edition of Isidore's *Etymologies* by W. M. Lindsey, published by Oxford University Press, Oxford, 1911, has been reproduced on the Internet, at: *http://penelope.uchicago. edu/Thayer/L/Roman/Texts/Isidore/home.html.* Site visited on September 20, 2007.

4. Max Sheler. *Ordo Amoris.* In: *Selected Philosophical Essays.* Translated, with an introduction by David R. Lachterman. Evanston, Ill.: Northwestern University Press, 1973, pp. 98 135.

5. A recent scholarly study of the story of the "devoured heart" in its different forms, to which I am indebted for much of the material in this section, was published in Spanish: Isabel de Riquer: *El Corazón Devorado. Una leyenda desde el siglo XII hasta nuestros días.* Madrid: Ediciones Siruela, 2007.

6. The Egyptian narrative is transcribed by Milad Doueihi in his erudite work on the symbolism of the heart: *Histoire Perverse du Coeur Humain.* Paris: Seuil, 1996, pp. 29–32. This book was published in English as *A Perverse History of the Human Heart.* Cambridge, Mass.: Harvard University Press, 1998.

7. Quoted by Isabel de Riquer, loc. cit., pp. 23–24.

8. Madame d'Aulnoy. *Mémoires de la Cour d'Espagne.* The Hague: Adrien Moetjens, 1691, pp. 108–109. For a wider discussion of the legend of the "devoured heart" in Spanish culture, see: John D. Williams: "Notes on the legend of the eaten heart in Spain." *Hispanic Review* XXVI (2) (April 1958): 91–98.

9. Isabel de Riquer, loc. cit.

10. Meyer Friedman and Gerald W. Friedland. "William Harvey and the Circulation of the Blood." Chapter 2 in *Medicine's Ten Greatest Discoveries.* New Haven: Yale University Press, 1998.

11. Quoted by Meyer Friedman and Gerald W. Friedland. Ibid.

12. William Harvey. "Of the abundance of blood passing through the heart and out the veins into the arteries, and of the circular motion of the blood." Chapter VIII in *De Motu Cordis*. I used the fine edition of *De Motu Cordis* edited by Geoffrey Keynes, from a copy of a limited edition contemporary with: William Harvey. *The Anatomical Exercises. De Motu Cordis and De Circulatione Sanguinis in English translation.* New York: Dover, 1995.

13. Robert A. Erickson. *The Language of the Heart, 1600–1750.* See chapter 2, entitled "The Phallic Heart: William Harvey's 'The Motion of the Heart' and 'The Republick of Literature.'" Philadelphia: University of Pennsylvania Press, 1997, pp. 61–88.

14. Ibid, pg. 76.

15. Giulia Sissa and Marcel Detienne. *La Vie Quotidienne des Dieux Grecs.* Paris: Hachette, 1989, pp. 261–264.

16. The quotation is from chapter XIV of Joris-Karl Huysmans's novel *Là-Bas.* I used the 1995 edition by Maxi-Poche, Classiques Français, Paris, pg. 222 (author's translation).

17. A record of the conversation between Peter Allinson, one of the patients, and Melissa Larner, writer and editor, was published in: James Peto (editor): *The Heart.* New Haven: Yale University Press, 2007 (hereinafter referred to as James Peto's *The Heart*), pp. 65–69.

18. Quoted by Ayesha Nathoo in: "The trasplanted heart. Surgery in the 1960s." Chapter 6 in James Peto's *The Heart*, pg. 163.

19. Ibid, pg. 165.

20. Ernest Cutz, Herrman Yeger, and Jin Pan. "Pulmonary Neuroendocrine Cell System in Pediatric Lung Disease: Recent Advances." *Pediatric and Developmental Pathology* 10 (6) (2007): 419–435.

21. Marc S. Penn and Earl E. Bakken. "Heart-brain medicine: Where we go from here and why." *Cleveland Clinic Journal of Medicine* 74 (supplement 1) (February 2007): S4–S6.

22. G. L. Engel. "Sudden and rapid death during psychological stress: Folklore or folk wisdom?" *Annals of Internal Medicine* 74 (1971): 771–782.

23. Martin A. Samuels. "'Voodoo' death revisited: The modern lessons of neurocardiology." *Cleveland Clinic Journal of Medicine* 74 (supplement 1) (February 2007): S8–S16.

24. J. Andrew Armour. "The little brain on the heart." Ibid, pp. S48–S51.

25. Ilan S. Wittstein. "The broken heart syndrome." Ibid, pp. S17–S22.

26. The pathology of the heart after severe mental stress is discussed and illustrated in the following articles: M. S. Cebelin and C. S. Hirsch. "Human stress cardiomyopathy: Myocardial lesions in victims of homicidal assaults without internal injuries." *Human Pathology* 11 (1980): 123–132; D. Pavin, H. Le Breton, and C. Daubert. "Human stress cardiomyopathy mimicking acute myocardial syndrome." *Heart* 78 (1997): 509–511; I. S. Wittsein, D. R. Thiermann, J. A. Lima, et al. "Neurohumoral features of myocardial stunning due to sudden emotional stress." *New England Journal of Medicine* 352 (2005): 539–548.